Alzheimer's A to Z

alzheimer's
a to z

SECRETS to SUCCESSFUL CAREGIVING

BY

JYTTE LOKVIG, BA, MA

Endless Circle Press

Published by ENDLESS CIRCLE PRESS

For information, please contact:
Endless Circle Press
228 Ojo de la Vaca
Santa Fe, NM 87508
(505)466-8195 or (575)466-8195

Second Printing

ISBN: 0-9710390-0-3

LIBRARY OF CONGRESS CATALOG CARD NUMBER: 2001089597

Publisher's Cataloging-in-Publication
Lokvig, Jytte.
    Alzheimer's A to Z : secrets to successful caregiving
/ Jytte Lokvig ; illustrations by the author. -- 1st ed.
    p. cm.
    Includes bibliographical references.
    LCCN: 2001089597
    ISBN: 0-9710390-0-3

    1. Alzheimer's disease—Popular works.
    2. Alzheimer's disease—Patients—Care—Popular works.
    I. Title.
    RC523.2.L65 2002   616.8'31
                        QBI01-200581

Illustrations by the author
(Any resemblance to real people is purely coincidental).

Cover Design by Joseph Loveria

Printed in the United States

Dedicated to my friend Bahtee, who gave me the inspiration and encouragement to write this book.

TABLE OF CONTENTS

Appendix

FOREWORD

In this new millennium the disorders of dementia will be more evident, with few people not touched by the effects of this debilitating disease. The increasing numbers of our aging population will place growing demands on society. None will be more challenging than the tasks of the caregiver with a loved one afflicted by a dementing illness.

On reading Alzheimer's A to Z, my staff responded with smiles of agreement and an enthusiastic "Yes--this is what is needed!" This wonderful resource, simply expressed and logically presented, inspires confidence in caregivers and loved ones while offering simple paths through the maze of daily challenges. Topics are organized for easy reference, allowing readers to quickly locate information as new situations arise.

Alzheimer's caregiving demands an empathy not always easily available. Those of us who have chosen Aged Care as a profession, especially in the sphere of dementia, have in the past relied on 'on the job' learning experiences to augment our knowledge, resources, and training. The key to understanding this confusing world is in how we communicate. Our results can create a secure, trusting, and often humorous environment. This timely book captures typical experiences and suggests workable solutions. It spells out the pitfalls, and realistically guides the frustrated with basic pointers in dealing with loved ones. Ms. Lokvig speaks from the heart with compassion for everyone afflicted with this complex disease, providing hope and confidence to those charged with the task of their care. Her message is one of acceptance, humility and love.

Catherine Wallace, RN
The New South Wales Executive of
the Australian Association of Gerontology
and Director of "Marian" Dementia Aged Care Facility
North Parramatta, Sydney, Australia

ACKNOWLEDGMENTS

This book is a labor of love, which could not have happened without my many friends with Alzheimer's and dementia, who over the years have taught me how to appreciate the smallest pleasures found in every new day. And my gratitude to all the many families who have so generously shared their experiences. Many persons contributed to this project and it's hard to single out any one. Heather Darden, Cecelia Davidson, Cookie Jordan, Arthur Silvers, and Kristin Slater: you patiently supported me throughout this project, letting me bounce ideas off of you at all hours of the day.

Damaris Ames, Deanna Bellinger, Mary Ellen Carroll, Glenn Chippindale, RN, Robert Margolin, Paula Petersen, and Archie Tew: I appreciate your generous input and sharing you expertise. And to Rockne Tarkington: You gave me the key to unlocking my voice.

Douglas Houston, Haven Lin-Kirk, and Gaston Lokvig: Thank you for your technical support.

Special thanks to Alexis Higginbotham. Your consistent feedback and discriminating editing were vital to the development of this book.

And most of all, my family: without your solid support and encouragement this book would have remained a dream.

PREFACE

Several years ago a friend asked me help out with her mother while she was away on an extended business trip. Her mother had Alzheimer's and needed someone to visit with her for a few hours a day.

I had read about Alzheimer's, of course, but had never met anyone with the disease. I had no idea what to expect. The first visit was a disaster. My new acquaintance greeted me sweetly enough, but she spent the entire visit worrying about who I was and what I was doing there. None of my attempts at conversation worked and I left feeling a complete failure. Determined to make this work, I decided to share my own interests with her and took her to one of my favorite art galleries. She was engrossed. From then on we visited galleries regularly and started making collages from the announcements that we'd picked up along the way. It wasn't long before she was creating on her own. And while she cut and pasted, we talked. We talked about our lives, loves, funny experiences, and some sad ones. Her stories were often disjointed and confused, but over time I pieced together a picture of her life. We became true friends.

Other families started coming to me for help and soon we were a whole group. We made music and art, wrote stories and discussed everything under the sun. We visited the library and museums, went to the movies and picnicked by the river.

I read everything I could find on Alzheimer's disease, but there was very little that helped me with my daily situations, so I had to find my own solutions. A person with Alzheimer's disease or dementia is not "sick" as such, but rather in an altered state of mind and still capable of having a rich life. It quickly became clear to me that my friends all thought of themselves as quite normal in a world that felt increasingly confusing to them.

I address the "normal" in everyone and work with their individual interests and needs. Together we invent the days as we go along. The goal is to have rich and fulfilling experiences, no matter how insignificant they might appear to others. The most special times are when we just talk. I mostly listen, because everyone needs an ear. I work with folks from diverse backgrounds, with different interests, temperaments, and all levels of dementia. I've found that certain attitudes, ways of communication, and approaches are consistently effective with everyone, regardless of the degree of impairment. Over the years I have shared these tools with families and care facilities with most satisfying results. I decided it was time to share them with you. This book is compiled from my own experiences and the situations that invariably come up for other caregivers.

Jytte Lokvig

INTRODUCTION

You've opened your heart and home to your Mom since she's been diagnosed with Alzheimer's and can no longer take care of herself. She's very angry at being uprooted from her own house, but you know that you've done the right thing. Your life is often in turmoil now and Mom's so resistant to your care that you've seriously considered placing her in a care facility, even if it means mortgaging your own house to pay for it.

Before you take such a drastic measure, consider using the tips outlined in this accessible A to Z guide to caregiving. We've compiled this book from actual experiences, using real problems and real solutions. The situations may not be identical to yours, but it's likely that they're similar enough that you can adapt them to suit your needs. We frequently refer to "Mom" and "Dad" in this book, though in fact you may be caring for your husband, wife, aunt, uncle, friend, partner, or client.

Taking care of a person with Alzheimer's is a major undertaking that should be shared, and you have the right to insist that family pitch in. Take advantage of all the local support that is available to you. The Alzheimer's Association holds support group meetings in most communities, and other government agencies can direct you to local programs that can give both you and Mom a respite. These same agencies can also help you later if you need to find a full-time care facility for her. You might have a full-time job and a full-time caregiver to help you out. In that case, it's very important that both you and your caregiver use this book.

The key to your success will be your overall attitude. Life with Mom will be much less stressful with minor adjustments to your vocabulary and approach. We often recommend that you take a deep breath before dealing with a particularly difficult situation. This gives you time to pull yourself together to face it. You'll get very good at deep breathing and your patience level will definitely increase. You'll learn to take things in stride and forgive yourself for slip-ups. You'll discover the small pleasures and joys in life with Mom so that the time spent with her will become enriched for both of you.

You can use our A to Z suggestions to aid you in exploring new avenues to reach Mom and to help her through this. She may not be able to express her feelings to you anymore, and she's most likely afraid and confused. Her world has gone topsy-turvy and she often has no idea where she is or who she is. If she lashes out at you in anger, she's probably trying to let you know just how frightened she really is. She needs you to be strong, calm, and reassuring. In the beginning you'll have to learn to ignore her outbursts and reassure her that she is loved and appreciated by you. The first few weeks are the most difficult, but with practice your reactions will become second nature.

In order to survive this caregiving experience with your heart intact, it's important to remember that the "stranger" who has replaced Mom is still a vital human being with a lot of love, laughter, and enjoyment left to live. It is by no means an easy path to take, but instead of mourning the loss of your Mom while she's still alive, celebrate the person she is now.

Hope sees the invisible, feels the intangible, and achieves the impossible.

-Anonymous

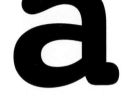

ACCEPTANCE

You've thought of Mom as your best friend for most of your adult life so when she needed it, it seemed so natural to open your home to her. You wouldn't have thought otherwise.

Now that you've accustomed yourself to the slower pace of life with Mom, all in all, things are going well. Then one day you wake her for breakfast and she behaves as if she has no idea who you are. She clutches her blanket in obvious terror as she screams at the top of her lungs at this "stranger" who has invaded her bedroom. She accuses you of keeping her prisoner and not letting her go back to her own house. You explain until you're blue in the face why she's now living with you. Mom sulks and you're filled with sadness and guilt. You try to comfort her but she keeps pulling away from you in her panic. Your heart breaks. Your own mother doesn't know who you are and you have no idea what to do.

"If you don't know who I am, Mom, then how can I recognize myself in your eyes?" You don't. The painful irony is that although we've always considered ourselves to be the center of our parents' universe, the reality is that long before we were ever born our parents had full lives with friends, relationships, and experiences that didn't revolve around us. Acknowledging that gives us a new understanding of who they are.

Mom may mistake you for her cousin, her second-grade teacher, or her college roommate, but it's obvious that she recognizes you as a person whom she trusts and loves. Your willingness to be accepted as these different people will give you the valuable opportunity to learn more about your Mom, not only who she was as your mother, but who she is as a human being, woman, friend, cousin, daughter, lover, teacher, wife.

ॐ

Dad's so different now from just a few years ago before the onset of his dementia. It's very hard to come to grips with the fact that the father you once knew will never return. Sometimes when he says or does something familiar, behaving just like his old self, you want to hang on to him to keep him from disappearing again. It's natural to grieve your loss, but at the same time try, for the sake of your own emotional survival, to learn to accept him as he is.

While it's a fact that Dad's dementia is never going to improve, it doesn't mean that he can't still be a meaningful person in your life. Take your caregiving experience one day at a time and set yourself reasonable goals. Appreciate small achievements: an easy bath time or a pleasant outing. And when you make it through a whole day without a hitch, celebrate your successes.

Don't be too hard on yourself, because the process of acceptance takes time. Even though Dad's not the same anymore, who he is now can be interesting, fun, and even lovable. Don't beat yourself up when you feel the sadness come over you. Instead, ask Dad for a big hug.

(Also: Comprehension, Empathy, Normal)

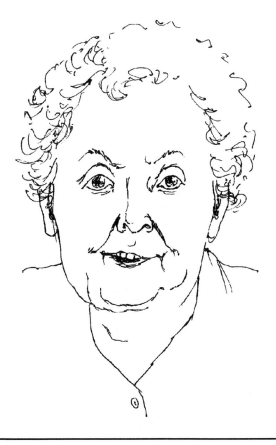

The old woman I shall become will be quite different from the woman I am now. Another I is beginning.

- George Sand

ACTIVITIES

Activities are essential to the mental wellbeing of everyone, and your husband is no exception. He may not be able to recall many of the things you do together, but the experiences still help him feel enriched and involved. As a successful caregiver, you'll discover a healthy balance between maintenance, such as showers and meals, and activities that he does by himself and with you that provide pleasure and personal fulfillment.

Retirement can be difficult for your husband. He doesn't have his job to give him a reason to get up in the morning and he misses the validation he felt from receiving a paycheck. Successful retirees find substitute activities to keep themselves stimulated and vital, but because of his dementia, your husband is not able to do this for himself. He needs you to help make things happen for him. This book contains ideas for games, group projects, excursions, and special activity areas at home. In the beginning it may take some extra effort on your part, but soon the result will be a happier man and an easier life for both of you.

The success of your husband's projects depends a lot on your attitude. No matter what his activity, it's important that you take it seriously. However uncomplicated the project might be, your attitude will give it legitimacy and importance.

He's been restless since breakfast. He needs something to do to help him get back to feeling good about himself. Begin by asking for his help:

"Excuse me, sweetie, are you busy right now? I sure could use your help. Let me show you. See this stack of catalogs? I can't make heads or tails of them. Could you help me sort them out, please? You've always been so good at that sort of thing."

After he agrees:
"Let's see . . . we have Time, Good Housekeeping, Forbes, and what's this? Oh, that's the new computer magazine we ordered. How do you suggest we do it?"

Wait for his suggestion and no matter what it is, let him know you think it's a good one. Encourage him to take the time necessary to reach his conclusion. It takes a lot of patience on your part, but in the process you are letting him know that you value his input and, in turn, you're affirming his feeling of self-determination. It's important that you do not talk to him like a child; he's demented but he's not stupid.

(Also: Exercise, Games, Kitchen, Outings, Projects, Reading, Personal Space, Singing)

If you don't like something, change it; if you can't change it, change the way you think about it.
- Mary Engelbreit

AFFECTION

"Dad, may I have a hug from you, please?"

Dad beams as he straightens his back and reaches out to hold you. For one brief moment you're six years old again, and he's your big, strong Daddy, who never let anything bad happen to you. You feel it and he feels it.

Dad has great difficulty with his speech these days so you're relying more and more on nonverbal communication. You've discovered that displays of affection like hugs, kisses, and handholding all seem to calm Dad down and make him more responsive to you. You make a point of touching and hugging him many times a day, but it's important that you occasionally ask for his permission:

"Dad, may I give you a hug?"

Or: "Dad, I really need a good hug right now. May I have one, please?"

And after the hug:
"Thank you, your hugs always make me feel so good."

Or: "May I give you a back rub?"

Or: "May I have a kiss, please?"

By asking for his consent, you're offering him a choice that helps boost his feeling of control over his life. He may surprise you by becoming much more cooperative and attentive.

(Also: Massage, Questions)

AGE

Age can be a touchy subject once we reach our forties or fifties, since growing old doesn't fit in very comfortably with our youth-conscious society. Aging can be hard on anyone, so why would anyone presume it's okay to exclaim to an elderly person, "You're 90, wow! How does it feel?" when we wouldn't dream of exclaiming, "You're 55, wow! How does it feel?"

Mom often becomes upset if people around her make a big deal about her "ripe old age," so you may have to intercede on her behalf. Professionals, such as doctors and nurses, may talk to you about Mom in her presence as if she doesn't understand a word. Age often comes up. She probably doesn't remember her actual age, but she may still relate being in her eighties or nineties as being "very old." That is a depressing thought.

Instead you can encourage a conversation about how old everyone feels inside, "in spirit." In these discussions, Mom most frequently recalls the events of her young adulthood or college days, which were times in her life when she felt the most empowered and independent.

(Also: Birthdays, Comprehension, Dignity, Empathy, Normal)

To know how to grow old is the masterwork of wisdom, and one of the most difficult chapters in the great art of living.
-Henri-Frederic Amiel

AGGRESSION

Mom suddenly lashes out, kicking you and screaming inco-
herently. Something has triggered her outburst. Before you
can deal with anything, you need to calm her down. In a firm
but gentle voice, say loudly enough to grab her attention,

"Mom, I can't understand what you are saying. Please lower
your voice so I can hear you. I want to help you."

Or, very loudly, "Mom, I LOVE YOU!"

Then if she seems receptive,

"May I have a hug? I need a hug, please?"

Once she's calmer, change her environment by taking her into
another room. As you sit her down, give her a hug, if she'll let
you, and say:

"Mom, I love you and it hurts me to see you this upset. I want
to help you. Can you tell me what's happening?"

"I want to go home. You're keeping me prisoner here! I don't
want to be here. I want to go home!"

Is she talking about the small apartment she lived in before
she came to live with you? Or does she mean your childhood
home or her own? Regardless, it serves no purpose while she
is in her current state of mind to remind her that her "home"
is now occupied by someone else. At other times she seems to
understands and accept this fact, but probably not now.

"Maybe we can go later, Mom, but I'm about to fix lunch and
you told me a few minutes ago that you were starved, so why
don't we eat lunch first?"

You have a leisurely lunch and after you've finished, you say: "May I have a hug, Mom? I'm so happy that you're in my life! Have I told you lately how glad I am that we're able to spend so much time together?"

In Public

You and Mom have just had a delightful lunch and now it's time to go home. You exit the restaurant and find yourself trying to steer her through the streaming mass of people walking along the sidewalk. Suddenly something spooks her. She yanks her arm away as she tries to pull out of your grip and screams:

"Help, call the police! Call the police! Help me, I'm being kidnapped!"

You're astounded as she pummels your arm with all her might because you had no idea she was capable of that kind of strength. Some people stop and stare while others quickly look away, not wanting to get involved. One person steps up to "help." Mom grabs his arm and falls into his embrace, giving you no choice but to release her. As you look up into the man's face, you're startled to find that he's glaring at you!

This is about as upsetting as anything that has happened so far. In the back of your mind the thought of nursing homes and restraints is taking shape and the idea is looking mighty good to you right now. Mom looks like a perfectly lucid and normal woman to strangers while you're so upset that you're probable looking like the wacky one at the moment. This man thinks you are a BAD person.

You're mortified. Take a deep breath and wait to speak until you can use a normal tone of voice, then calmly turn to the stranger:

"Thanks so much for helping me with Mother. It can get pretty difficult for Mom in these crowds because her Alzheimer's sometimes makes her feel claustrophobic. I appreciate your concern."

For once you might actually need to speak to Mom in a patronizing tone in order to get your point across to the "rescuer." Unfortunately most people assume that's the way caregivers are always supposed to communicate:

"Mother, we need to go home now. Be a dear and say thank you to the nice man."

Once you're finally away from the crowd, the real challenge is not to be angry with her. She most likely has already forgotten the incident. For your own sanity, you may need to get it off your chest, so call a person from your Alzheimer's support group, a good friend, or a family member so you can share your experiences and feelings.

(Also: Conversations, Diversions, Empathy, Going Home, Identification, No!, Safe Return)

Would those of you who say it can't be done, stop bothering those of us who are doing it

             -Anonymous

AGITATION

You had been very apprehensive about moving your Dad into your spare room, but now that he's lived with you for a while, it's been fine. Dad's been easygoing and undemanding, and you've enjoyed his company far more than you'd expected. Lately, however, he's been completely different – angry, short-tempered, and uncooperative. He'll lash out at you one minute and withdraw into despondency the next. You've tried a lot of the suggestions in this book, but nothing seems to help. It's been difficult and confusing for you. It's likely there's a good cause for Dad's feelings that has absolutely nothing to do with you. Consider meeting with his doctor if you suspect that Dad's problem might be physical.

- Has anything changed in his physical life lately?
- Is he reacting to medications?
- Was anything changed in his room recently?
- Are his shoes too tight? Do his clothes bother him?
- If he's wearing a brief, is it uncomfortable or wet?
- Have you noticed a sudden decline in his comprehension or speech? (He may be aware of this and may need extra support from you.)
- Has his physical condition changed lately, i.e., constipation, dental problems, or dehydration?
- Has his hearing or sight changed lately?

(Also: Aggression, Diversions, Environment)

If I knew what I was so anxious about,
I wouldn't be so anxious.
                    -Mignon McLaughlin

ALTERNATIVE REMEDIES

Consult with your physician before using any medicine, including alternative medicine. Today many doctors are supportive of alternative healing methods. However if your doctor is not comfortable with this issue, you may want to change to a holistic health provider.

Bilberry acts as a diuretic and urinary tract antiseptic. It may be one of the few substances that can halt macular degeneration. It is also helpful with night blindness and cataracts.

Ginkgo biloba is derived from the ancient ginkgo tree. It is primarily used to treat the ailments of the elderly, especially to improve mental function and promote circulation. Ginkgo biloba has been used for centuries in China to combat aging. In Europe studies have shown remarkable results. A few studies are under way in this country.

Ginseng is the most widely used medicine in China where it's known as a longevity tonic. For over a hundred years it has also been used in Europe. This herb is useful for lack of energy, stress, circulatory problems, and it enhances the immune system. It's believed to protect against radiation damage and shrink cancer tumors.

Gotu kola is good for heart and liver health as well as cardiovascular and circulatory functions. It also stimulates the nervous system and improves poor appetite and mental function.

Rosemary aids with circulatory problems and irregular blood pressure. It also has anti-cancer and anti-tumor properties.

St. Johns Wort helps with nerve pain and depression. It is a good alternative to prescription antidepressants. However, do not use without consulting your physician. This herb sometimes has adverse effects in people who suffer from serious arthritis or an immune system deficiency.

Coenzyme Q10 is a vitamin-like substance found naturally in the body where it declines as we age. It's a potent antioxidant with effects resembling those of vitamin E, only more powerful. It has been prescribed for years in Japan for millions of people with heart disease. Coenzyme Q10 is a strong immune system booster especially beneficial for circulation and tissue oxygenation, and is critical to cell growth. It's also used to treat mental dysfunction such as schizophrenia and Alzheimer's disease. Coenzyme Q10 is oilsoluble and best when taken with oily or fatty foods. Look for a liquid or oil form with a small amount of vitamin E added.

Hyperzine (HupA) is thought to work similarly to the prescription drugs tacrine and donepezil, but with less toxic risk.

Melatonin is a hormone that provides protection for every cell in our bodies. It has been found to have amazing abilities to protect against a wide array of disorders.

(Also: Dementia, Diet, Vitamins)

Never go to a doctor whose office plants have died.
-Erma Bombeck

ALZHEIMER'S DISEASE

Mom has had "senior moments" for several years. She'd forget names, misplace her keys, and mix up the dates of her children's birthdays, but recently her behavior and personality have changed. She's getting very confused and quite agitated. You fear she's developing Alzheimer's disease. Before you jump to this conclusion remember that there are many correctable conditions that exhibit Alzheimer's-like symptoms, so it's important for Mom to undergo a thorough physical examination.

Alzheimer's disease is named after Dr. Alois Alzheimer, a German neuropathologist, who identified the disease in 1906. A patient at a local mental institution had exhibited severe dementia for ten years before her death at age 55. During the autopsy on her brain, Dr. Alzheimer found tangled nerve cells and plaque deposits that he believed to be the cause of her dementia. Alzheimer's disease is the term for a specific deterioration of nerve clusters in the brain. These clusters become calcified and tangled, rendering them ineffective.

At this time there are between four and six million victims of Alzheimer's disease in this country, of whom approximately one million live in care facilities. With the aging of our population, these numbers are expected to increase dramatically. Research into the condition has also increased, but we continue to have many more questions than answers. Some medications on the market can ease or delay symptoms for some folks. There are some promising developments in the search for a vaccine. One substance appears to dissolve existing plaques in lab animals.

Progression. Alzheimer's disease begins with a loss of short-term memory, progressing through confusion, loss of cognitive function to a complete loss of all bodily functions. These disorders usually progress very slowly, so nothing is going to change drastically in Mom's condition anytime soon. In the meantime the best approach is to work on a change in lifestyle. Above all, don't panic. Following the ideas in this book can help improve life for both of you.

Causes

What causes Alzheimer's is still unknown and there is no known cure. Science is looking at genetic connections, biochemical changes, and environmental factors, such as head trauma in the patient's past, alcohol abuse, and toxins.

The Genetic Connection. Research has identified three chromosomes apparently responsible for early onset Alzheimer's (people in their 30s to 50s): Chromosomes 1, 14, and 21. (Chromosome 21 appears to be responsible for Down's syndrome as well.) Together these three chromosomes account for only about 5% of all Alzheimer's cases. A fourth, APOE4 (Chromosome 19.) has been showing up in 65% of all Alzheimer's patients studied.

At this point, there are no explanations for why some people develop Alzheimer's and others don't. Even if your parent has Alzheimer's disease with genetic causes there's no guarantee that you'll get it.

The Protein Connection. Numerous studies show an unusually high accumulation of amyloid beta protein in Alzheimer's brains as well as another protein named Tau. The greater the degree of dementia, the higher the levels of these proteins.

These are important discoveries in the search for more accurate tests, vaccines, and antidotes for the disease once it has set in.

The Folate and Choline Connections. There appears to be a correlation between a deficiency in folate and Alzheimer's disease. It is often found in connection with a deficiency of vitamin B12. Unfortunately this condition is not reversible once the disease has developed. Folate is found in legumes, salmon, tuna, citrus fruit, and root vegetables. (Cooking destroys folate.) Vitamin B12 is found only in animal foods such as milk, eggs, and most meat, especially liver.

Choline is crucial to the health of nerve transmitters in the brain and other organs. Some research is showing that serious choline deficiency is common in Alzheimer's victims. It is accepted by the health community that choline deficiency impairs the nervous system and brain function as well as the digestive system and blood pressure. Choline is found in meat, egg yolks, legumes, soybeans, and whole grain cereals.

The Aluminum Connection. Four times the normal amount of aluminum deposits is found in Alzheimer's brains upon autopsy. There's disagreement among researchers as to the significance of this. You may want to take precautions anyway and avoid excessive exposure to the metal. Aluminum is found in most deodorants, many douches, buffered aspirin, most shampoos, antacids, and of course aluminum cookware. There's also aluminum in many food products such as cake mixes, frozen dough, and sliced processed cheese. Juice cartons are lined with aluminum and many other beverages also come in aluminum cans.

Environmental Toxins. There appears to be correlation between the use of herbicides (weed killers) and insecticides (bug sprays) and the development of Alzheimer's. Another study shows that Alzheimer's is more prevalent among persons who have been exposed excessively to household cleaners.

Tests

After Mom has had her thorough physical and it has been ascertained that her dementia is not caused by a reversible and correctable condition, her doctor should refer her to a neurologist, who will give Mom verbal memory tests and likely order a MRI (Magnetic Resonance Imaging) or CAT scan. Doctors caution against testing for APOE4. At this point the only reliable test for this genetic connection is a spinal tap. Research is under way for a simple skin test.

Vaccines

There is cautious optimism about an Alzheimer's vaccine currently under development. Researchers have identified a substance that successfully prevents the formation of plaques in aged lab animals. It even shows signs of dissolving existing plaques. Tests have been started on people. So far there are no serious side effects in human subjects. It will take several years to learn if these substances are effective as vaccines. Several prominent leaders within the Alzheimer's community express caution, reminding us that many good results with animal subjects from other promising vaccines (such as those for diabetes) have not been effective with people.

Medications

Alzheimer's Medication. Three medications are available for Alzheimer's: Cognex (tacrine,) Aricept (donepezil,) and Exelon (rivastigmine tartrate.) These drugs may be of benefit during the early stages of Alzheimer's by delaying the progression of symptoms. However they do not prevent or cure the disease. They may have serious side effects such as gastric upset and liver damage (tacrine.) Before you commit Dad to one of these drugs, be sure that you familiarize yourself with possible side effects, interactions, and other risks.

Estrogen. Most studies indicate that estrogen replacement therapy may protect women from developing Alzheimer's or delay the onset of the disease. Starting estrogen after the onset of Alzheimer's has shown no therapeutic effect.

NSAIDs. Ibuprofen (e.g. Advil, Motrin) has been suggested in some literature for Alzheimer's disease. However, leading experts caution against the liberal use of NSAIDs in the elderly, because of the risk of serious side effects such as gastric injuries (GI bleeds).

Research suggests that ibuprofen may have a preventive effect in moderate doses of 800 mg a day. It may delay the very early stages of Alzheimer's disease, but it's not recommended once the disease is in progress. Side effects (GI bleeds) show up in 15-20% of people taking chronic daily doses of 600-1200 mg. There's also a concern about interactions with other medication. You might want to consider alternatives, such as vitamin supplements, herbal remedies, and diet, even though the effects may not be as dramatic.

(Also:Alternative Remedies, Dementia, Diet, Normal, Vitamins)

Optimism is the faith that leads to achievement.
Nothing can be done without hope or confidence.
-Helen Keller

ANGER

Dad used to be very strict with you when you were a child, scolding you when you needed it and sometimes when you did not. Now you're finding yourself biting your tongue when he does or says some of the very things that he used to reprimand you for. It's hard not to give him a taste of his own medicine.

You're getting very good at deep breathing, aren't you? When these very natural resentments and feelings of anger arise in you, take a deep breath and put your feelings aside until you can share them with a good friend, a family member, or your Alzheimer's support group. Hopefully your siblings are available to listen so you can share some of the scary, not-yet-resolved feelings about Dad that might surface for each of you, even though at times the family might just want to avoid the subject altogether.

◎

Mom's been agitated and upset all day and you're exhausted. Nothing you've tried has been able to calm her down. You've been so patient that you feel like your halo must be glowing, but nothing seems to help. She's been sobbing that she wants to "go home." You manage to distract her by getting her involved in her personal space "office," but it only lasts ten minutes and then she starts interrupting you all over again. You have all this housework and laundry to do; how the heck are you ever going to get it done? Although you realize that Mom can't help how she behaves, part of you is so sure that she's doing this just to annoy you; she knows exactly what she's doing and she just wants to drive you crazy!

These are the times when you feel trapped by your circumstances. Will this ever end? You resist the impulse to shake

Mom back to her senses. Take a deep breath and, if you need to, go outside by yourself for a few minutes. So what if you don't wash the dishes today? Nothing is more important than you and Mom at this particular time. After you have collected yourself, focus your attention on Mom:

"Mom, I'm so sorry I've been so distracted this afternoon. I forgot for a while what's really important. And you know what that is? You and me! How would you like to go for a drive to the bakery? We'll buy some donuts and have a celebration; doesn't that sound good?"

You're having this celebration as much for yourself as for Mom. As soon as you're feeling better, she'll probably calm down again because her moods tend to reflect yours. This dual responsibility of physical and mental caregiving can be an enormous burden on you and can aggravate your feelings of anger. If these feelings of anger or rage happen only occasionally, you can regard them as a natural part of the caregiving process. However, if they start to happen so frequently that they're interfering with your wellbeing, consider talking to a professional, like a therapist or a counselor, or even a psychiatrist. You aren't weak or crazy if you go to outside sources for assistance. As you know by now, taking care of Mom is difficult and emotionally draining at times. Any support and advice you can get will help you stay sane through the rough moments and ultimately benefit both you and her.

(Also: Counseling, Home Help, Respite, Support Groups)

Happiness walks on busy feet.
                    -Kitte Turmell

APPETITE

Dad's appetite has changed. Sometimes he'll barely touch his lunch, while at other times it seems he won't stop eating. His dementia may actually affect his feelings of hunger and satiation, so he has no sense of when and how much to eat. Questions to ask yourself in this situation:

- Is his medication affecting his appetite?
- Is he having elimination problems?
- Is he having dental problems?
- Is he suffering from aches and pains?
- Is he getting good exercise?
- Is his spirit otherwise good?
- Is he showing signs of depression?
- Is he forgetting how to use eating utensils?

If these aren't problem areas, it may be a result of his Alzheimer's and you can continue as you have been, but try to develop some adaptability in your mealtime preparations and have fun with them. If Dad is ravenous one day, then cook him an enormous breakfast, and if the next day he's only interested in snacks, let him snack. Why do we have to do three squares every day, anyway? In the meantime, you can monitor his overall food consumption to ensure that he's getting his dietary requirements, adding vitamins and supplements when necessary. Discuss his diet with his doctor at his next physical.

(Also: Depression, Eating, Exercise)

Just trust yourself, then you will know how to live.
-Johann Wolfgang von Goethe

ATTITUDE

Alzheimer's disease has changed Mom's personality. She often does or says things that would have been totally out of character before she developed the disease. You may occasionally have a strong urge to shake her, hoping to bring her back to her senses, but you know that this would only aggravate the situation further. She cannot control her moods or feelings and more than ever she needs your support and acceptance. Sometimes it's difficult to control your own reactions, but you're constantly reminded that Mom mirrors your moods through her behavior.

There are times when you want to fly off the handle, but you control yourself with deep breathing. And if things get really bad and you think you may explode, go to another room or outside for a break. No matter what happens, try to remember that this is Alzheimer's disease and Mom is no longer in control of her behavior. However, you can influence her with your attitude. Decide what is really important at the moment. You often have to set aside your old ideas of what is proper and concentrate on Mom's needs from her perspective. If Mom is very agitated, your unruffled demeanor will help to subdue her. You may have to fake your initial reaction, because it can be very hard to accept that your mother can behave like this. After she has settled down again, use one of your effective diversions to get her into a positive state of mind.

You will find yourself changing your notions of what's important and your focus will turn to the enjoyment of sharing small everyday pleasures with Mom. And don't forget that humor and a lighthearted attitude will get you over many hurdles. Keep your humorous comment to things that she finds funny.

There will be times when she either does or says something sweetly funny. Hard as it may be at the moment, make sure you never laugh at her.

Begin each day with an upbeat greeting:

"Good morning to you, good morning to you . . . (to the tune of Happy Birthday). . . We're going to have a special day today! Let's start with a good breakfast. Breakfast is the most important meal of the day! That's what my Mom always said . . .. Oh, that's right, you are my Mom!"

Use encouraging remarks throughout the day to reinforce these good feelings:

"I'm so glad you thought of this."

Or: "We are having such a good day, aren't we?"

Or: "I'm so happy we can share this. It's so much better when we're doing this together."

Or: "I can't think of anything I'd rather be doing today."

Or: "Aren't we lucky that we have each other?"

You'll want to take care of yourself. Take time out with respite care assistance and the support of friends and family.

And try to maintain your sense of humor, because sometimes it's the only thing that keeps you from going completely crazy.

What often frustrates you is the attitude of others, so you have become an advocate for Mom. In public places you have learned to ignore the occasional insensitive stare. You're becoming her spokesperson when it comes to dealing with the outside world and you stand up on her behalf when she's confronted with patronizing or demeaning remarks or behavior from strangers.

As you go through this book, you'll find that the central theme is maintaining a positive attitude. It's not always easy, but by using a lighthearted approach to your daily situations, you'll discover that Mom often responds more favorably. Life becomes much easier for both of you.

(Also: Acceptance, Baby Talk, Conversations, Dignity, Diversions, Empathy, Normal, Questions, Reactions)

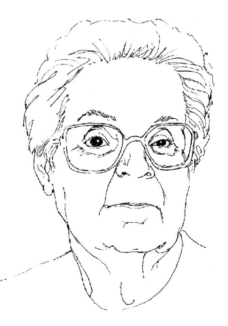

A happy person is not a person in a certain set of circumstances, but rather a person with a certain set of attitudes.

-Hugh Downs

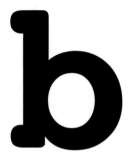

BABY TALK

You and Mom are out for an afternoon stroll, when you bump into an old acquaintance of yours. She's an effusive personality that bubbles uncontrollably. She beams at you like a spotlight, as she gushes,

"Oh, you and your mother are out for a little walk?"

She turns to Mom and pats her arm patronizingly as she gushes some more:

"Isn't that sweet of your son to take his Mommy out for walkies! Don't you look cute today, Dearie? What a sweet dress, just precious on you."

The look on Mom's face says it all: she is confused and upset. You'll have to do something. You could give this woman some of her own rude medicine:

"Well, Dahling, what brings you out into this revealing daylight? I must say that old dress still looks good on you!"

However, it's uncomfortable for you to use this kind of snide remark, and this person is probably too self-absorbed to get the point anyway.

Instead, tell her in plain English:

"Mom is a mature adult. She does not appreciate it when people talk to her in baby talk."

There are some people who resort to baby talk any time they encounter someone whom they perceive as weak or ill. They don't know how degrading it is to the person to whom they're talking, let alone how idiotic they make themselves sound when they talk that way. To speak in this manner to anyone but a baby, or perhaps a lover, is insulting, demeaning, and just plain rude. The most difficult situations are often with the most well meaning people, who don't realize that their tone of voice is patronizing.

If someone starts baby talking or cooing with Mom, you can kindly, but firmly interrupt with:

"I'm sorry, but my Mother relates best to a normal adult voice."

(Also: Attitude, Comprehension, Conversations, Dignity, Normal)

It's always something.
-Roseanne Roseannedanna (Gilda Radner)

BATHROOM

Toilet Coaching

It's important that Mom continues to use the toilet by herself for as long as possible. If it's necessary for you to supervise, remain calm and straightforward as you coach her through the motions:

"Let's use the toilet now, before we go out. You go first; I'll go after you. We can share a flush and save two-and-a-half gallons of water!"

You can gently direct her if she hesitates or seems confused about her clothes or the toilet itself:

"Here's the toilet (as you point to the toilet). Pull your pants and underwear down to your knees. There. Now you can sit down on the toilet. Let me give you a hand."

She may need guidance or physical assistance, so you want to be careful in the way you word your comments, so she can't answer, "No."

"Here's the toilet, would you like me to help you?"

"No."

Instead, use a remark that doesn't call for any answer:

"Here's the toilet. I'll give you a hand."

If you can, sit on the tub or a chair next to her and chat, then ask her if she has finished peeing or if she needs to have a "BM," or whatever term is familiar to her. Hand her the toilet tissue when she's finished and talk her through her motions:

"Here's some tissue to wipe with. Go ahead and wipe yourself down there."

You may need to demonstrate on yourself:

"See, this is how you do it. There, finished! Great! After you've pulled up your underwear and pants, it's my turn to pee."

Have her stay in the bathroom with you or keep the door open as you pee, so she'll be reassured to see that you go through the same motions. Using the toilet is a perfectly natural function. You'll build trust and confidence by sharing the experience with her. whenever you can.

❧

One morning as you're helping Mom get dressed, you notice that her nails are coated in a brown substance. It dawns on you that she has been scratching her anus. Maybe she can't figure out how to use the toilet paper anymore, or maybe she's constipated and has been trying to free herself of her stool. This is not unusual behavior for Alzheimer's patients. In the future, make it a point to check Mom's hands discreetly after she's used the toilet. You can use Handi-wipes to wipe her bottom and hands before you help her finish washing up:

"Let's see, Mom, we'd better wash this brown stuff off your hands. I'll run some water for you and you can let your hands soak for a minute. Might as well let the water do the work, right? Now you want to use some of this soap. There, you're as good as new!"

If this problem persists, talk to her doctor about getting her on a regimen of stool softener, fiber supplement, and increased liquid intake. You might also have her checked for hemor-rhoids, which can make elimination troublesome.

Bath Time
Everything had been going so well. You'd gotten quite adept at helping Mom with bathing, shampooing, and drying off. Suddenly one afternoon she lashes out at you, losing her tem-per and calling you names.

As Mom grows more dependent on you and others, she feels her self-determination slipping away. There are few activities left that allow her some semblance of control: bathing, eating, and dressing. Mom needs to feel some autonomy, but first she needs to calm down and feel safe with you again. Take her into another room and talk about something else for a while, or read the newspaper with her for until she is feeling more relaxed.

Before you decide to tackle bath time again, ask yourself:
• Does she really need a bath today?
• How frequently did she bathe in the past?

Most Americans bathe or shower daily, but she's from a gen-eration that bathed only when necessary. You might want to consider bathing her once or twice a week instead of every day. She may have very strong feelings about the time of day that she customarily takes her bath. For instance, did she usu-ally take her bath on Saturday mornings?

She may not remember what the bathing or showering proce-dure is, so when you ask her if she wants to take a bath, her first impulse may be to refuse firmly so she doesn't have to tackle all those things that seem scary and uncertain to her.

You decide to change your approach. Instead of asking her, try this alternative scenario:

"Mom, let me help you up."

"Why?"

"Come, I'll show you."

If she resists, talk about something unrelated while you help her out of her chair. Continue talking to her as you casually lead her to the bathroom. When you get there, you say:

"Yesterday, when we went to the store, you bought a wonderful new shampoo. You told me you wanted to try it today, so I'm going to turn on the shower for you so you can use it on your hair. I'll be glad to help you with your shower."

"I don't need a shower! I'm not dirty!"

"Oh, I know you're not dirty, but today's Saturday and that's your favorite shower day. Here we are! Here, smell this great shampoo. Your hair is going to smell so good, isn't it?"

Talk her step by step into the shower and onto the shower stool. After she's seated, turn on the water and let her feel the water stream from the hand-held shower. Keep adjusting it until she's pleased with the temperature. Patiently and cheerfully, coach her through the process. You'll want to encourage her to do as much as she can by herself. After she's dressed, reinforce how good she looks and how sweet her hair smells. Then you celebrate:

"Let's have a cup of tea and a chocolate chip cookie. How does that sound?"

As you relax with her, share an intimate conversation. By creating a relaxed environment, you're establishing bath time as a positive experience. If you stick to a routine that includes this comfortable connection, you'll build up trust and minimize problems down the road.

Keep a variety of soaps, shampoos, and towels on hand, and take shopping excursions to buy a new shampoo or soap. If you encourage her to make the selection, then later you can honestly admire her excellent choice.

ॐ

Tip! If Mom has trouble finding or using the toilet paper holder, get a standing paper towel holder, set it on the counter or on the floor next to the toilet and use it for toilet tissue. It's bigger and easier to see. Also, Mom may not be familiar with liquid soap, so keep a regular bar of soap at the sink.

(Also: Coaching, Compliments, Home Safety, No!, Questions)

There must be quite a few things a hot bath won't cure, but I don't know many of them.

-Sylvia Plath

BIRTHDAYS

You're hosting a party for Dad's birthday, complete with balloons, ice cream, and cake with lots of candles. Many of your friends have come to help celebrate. One of the guests cheerfully, but insensitively, exclaims,

"Wow, you are 91! How does that feel?"

Dad probably doesn't remember his chronological age, because nobody "feels" a certain age. Think about it. You feel tired. You feel energetic. You feel ill. But you don't "feel" a particular age. If anything, we relate age to wellbeing out of habit. "I feel a hundred, I am so tired!" or "I feel great today, positively like a teenager!"

Dad looks stricken and confused. Ninety-one is very old! Even a person with dementia knows that! You quickly go to his side, put your arms around him and cheerfully say,

"Dad, we are having a birthday party for you today. Which birthday would you like to celebrate?"

He enthusiastically replies,

"Twenty-eight!"

That's the birthday you'll be celebrating.

(Also: Age, Humor)

Beautiful young people are acts of nature,
but beautiful old people are works of art.
-Anonymous

BODY LANGUAGE

Mom may have a hard time expressing herself. You're becoming accustomed to observing her more subtle gestures and expressions in order to anticipate her needs and feelings.

Mom looks distracted as she pats the sides of her pants. You reach for a tissue and hand it to her as she smiles gratefully and blows her nose. She has trouble remembering words for common items, but fortunately you have become familiar with much of her body language. She does a certain little squirm when she needs the toilet, gives a unique twist of her mouth when she's thirsty, and has a distant look in her eyes that says it's nap time.

You're in the car and Mom's fidgety with a faraway look, so you say,

"You look as if you're hot. I think we should open the window, don't you?"

She mumbles and nods. As you go through the motions, describe what you are doing:

"I push a button over here to roll down your window. Magic, huh? That's better, isn't it? The fresh air sure smells good, doesn't it? You'll let me know if that is too windy, won't you?"

You know that chances are pretty slim that she'll be able to let you know. She may not be able to express it, but you give her a feeling of control whenever you notice how she feels. You learn to watch her out of the corner of your eye to make sure she's doing all right.

As you're becoming increasingly attuned to Mom's nonverbal communication, a private language develops between the two of you. The unexpected bonus is that you often feel closer to her as you learn to interpret these subtle signs of communication. Your favorite reaction from her is the twinkle in her eye when you suggest listening to Madama Butterfly, or a good story, or a drive in the car.

(Also: Empathy, Pain, Walking)

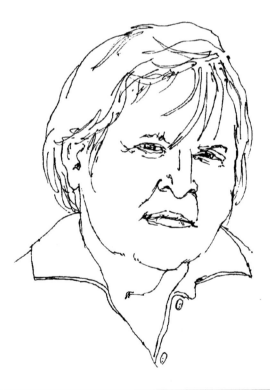

Love involves a peculiar unfathomable combination
of understanding and misunderstanding.
            -Diane Arbus

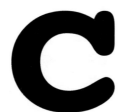

CARE FACILITIES

Most of us pay little attention to long-term care facilities until the need arises. Even if you may never have to face the possibility with Dad, it's a good idea to familiarize yourself now with the choices available in your community.

"In Dad's shoes, would I want to live here?"

Memory impaired folks are not sick as such and they don't need a hospital-like setting. The best Alzheimer's homes are designed with the comforts and atmosphere of a private home and the adaptations necessary for this special population. So, as you take the grand tour, look at it through Dad's eyes. Many facilities will spend fortunes on the décor in order to impress you, the "buyer." But as you well know, after a couple of days even the most esthetically conscious of us becomes oblivious to the wallpaper. What remains most important is good personal interaction between staff and residents and an environment of positive stimulation for the residents.

Categories

Talk to your local Ombudsman's office or request lists of facilities from your local agencies on aging. Ask questions, get opinions, and learn what your state requirements are for different types of facilities.

Independent living: Minimal personal care, unlicensed, unregulated. Usually apartment-type complexes with dining room and laundry facilities. Some meals and light housekeeping are usually included in monthly fees.

Assisted living: Some personal care, usually state licensed. Included in monthly fees should be meals, personal hygiene, housekeeping, and laundry. Most assisted-living facilities have resident nurses to supervise and dispense medication.

Nursing homes: Full nursing care, federally regulated, and state licensed. Medicaid eligible.

Alzheimer's homes: Full care for special-needs residents, state licensed. In some states they are Medicaid eligible.

Physical Environment

Large or small, the best Alzheimer's facilities are "user-friendly" homes. The attitude of management will emphasize the residents' quality of life. This can be hard to detect on a brief visit. You want the place to be attractive, but ask yourself: Is this place designed for the residents or is it designed for visitors like yourself? The furniture, color, and decorations should appear to be chosen for the pleasure and comfort of the residents, not to impress outsiders. Is the furniture especially selected for the comfort of the elderly, easy to get in and out of, while still looking attractive? Do the residents have free access to all the major living areas, indoors and out?

Is there evidence of celebration of the residents' individuality? You'll want to see signs of creativity and fun: books, games, flowers (albeit silk flowers), texture, and residents' art works displayed with respect and pride. Music and television should be for the pleasure of the residents. Room temperature comfort is important, around 75 degrees. Elderly folks are often cold, simply because they don't move around a lot.

Examine the promotional material and listen to the presentations made by the marketing people. The best facilities will put the emphasis on the mental well being of residents with special features like gardens, pets, music, and a variety of daily activities.

• Individual apartments or rooms should be attractively decorated and personalized as much as space allows. Shared rooms still offer privacy.

• The bathrooms are clean, spacious, handicap accessible, and have proper safety equipment. The bathrooms are plentiful and easy to find?

• The furnishings in common areas are comfortable, attractive, and arranged for socializing and activities. The public areas of the building offer residents a variety of cozy corners.

• The atmosphere of the facility is like that of a large home, not a hospital.

Residents
The residents should be dressed in clean, comfortable clothes appropriate to the time of day. You should witness frequent and positive interaction between staff and the residents. For example, if a staff member passes a resident in the process of doing her work, does she acknowledge the resident with a greeting, even if it's a simple "Hi!"?

The residents appear to be comfortable and content and interact to the best of their ability.

The artful grouping of furniture encourages conversations and socializing, and wheelchair residents are positioned closely to each other, making it easier for them to talk. There are obvious attempts to create social situations for the residents. Magazines, books, and photos are close at hand.

Staff
Staff members are pleasant, confident, and at ease when you talk to them. You observe them interact with residents in normal conversational tones, without condescending baby talk. They should handle agitated residents with calm, gentle diversions, without reprimands.

Request the number of staff who work directly with residents. Six residents to each staff member is a decent ratio. Ask about special qualifications of the staff, such as CNA (Certified Nurse's Assistant). Request a schedule of in-service subjects and development workshops, especially Alzheimer's training. Are they mandatory for the entire staff, anybody who has contact with residents? Inquire about contract employees. Contract employees have no benefits such as paid vacations and health care/medical coverage. It is a good indication of a facility's level of commitment to its staff.

As management does to staff, staff does to residents.

Activities

Request copies of menus and calendars of activities.

Menus reflect a nutritious, well-rounded diet that includes plenty of fruit and vegetables, which are also served as snacks throughout the day along with juices and water.

Indoor and outdoor activities include a variety of exercise programs and group events centered on music, art, and intellectual stimulation, with opportunities for individual creative expression.

The activities are tailored to the residents' interests and ability levels. If the facility has a diverse population, the programs accommodate the various levels, interests, and abilities of its residents.

Discuss with the activity director the unofficial activities beyond the scheduled arts and crafts programs. It's desirable to have a variety of routines open to resident participation: setting tables, assisting with cooking, folding laundry, sorting books, watering flowers, feeding resident animals, etc.

If the day comes when you must move Dad into a facility, as for its criteria in placing residents and assess the qualifications of those making the determination. Placing an individual having only slight dementia into a facility for seriously afflicted Alzheimer's residents can have devastating effects. It's also true that being placed with more highly functioning residents may further aggravate a very demented person's condition. Many facilities will gladly give you an "evaluation" of your parent, but be aware that some may be more interested in filling a bed than in giving you an accurate assessment. Get a second opinion, either from your local advocate for the aged or from a trusted physician with a specialty in geriatrics.

When you have tentatively chosen a place, request time to observe the facility's operations on your own. Spend enough time for the staff to get used to your presence and therefore go about their normal business. That way you are more likely to find out what Dad will really be living with. Sit in on activity sessions and eat a meal or two there. Observe the staff. Do they allow residents plenty of time to eat their meals and are they sensitive to individual needs, such as guiding one person with eating utensils and not offering all the courses of a meal at once, which can lead to a person to feel overwhelmed and confused? Spend some time with residents. Note their general mental and physical wellbeing. Does the staff talk to the residents often and with respect and dignity? Is a television on constantly? Do television and radio programs appear to be chosen for the enjoyment of the residents or does the staff make selections for their own pleasure?

Is the facility a comfortable "home"? Would you want to spend days on end in the "common room"? Is there ample open space and outdoor areas for walks, games, or picnics? What kind of intellectual stimulation is offered? Are there group and individual activities? What is the staff's attitude in general? How available is the staff to you? You'll want to share with them what you've learned from your experiences with Dad and you may want to give them a copy of this book for reference.

Good luck! And remember that even if you find the perfect facility, it's imperative that you still remain the center of Dad's life. Visit often, share meals with him, participate in conversations with his friends there, and take him on outings as much as possible.

(Also: Environment, Transitions)

All serious daring starts from within.
-Eudora Welty

CELEBRATIONS

Mom took great pride in her special Christmas cookies. The recipe had been handed down for generations and included a secret ingredient. Now she's no longer sure what kind of cookies they were, but she will still describe the process in minute detail.

Human beings thrive on ritual. All cultures have major holidays: Feast Day, Chanukah, Kwanzaa, Ramadan, New Years, or Christmas. Cookies, decorations, candles, feasting, and presents. All at once! No wonder this is a magic time.

Who says you can't celebrate Christmas in July or April? Put up the lights; bake cookies, light candles, and wrap presents with colorful ribbons. Your family may need some coercing to sing Christmas carols on a hot summer's day. Once you have adjusted yourself to this topsy-turvy world, you're all guaranteed to have a wonderful time.

You can create new rituals and celebrations anytime you want. You can have a "Friendship Party" to celebrate your living together. "First Day of Spring Party" and then a "We Cleaned out the Dresser Party" can follow a "Second Day of Spring Party." At other times you can make small daily celebrations by dressing up the kitchen with a special tablecloth, a bouquet of flowers, and a plate of goodies. You may want to add a surprise gift now and then. You can keep a stash of gift-wrapped boxes in a closet for just such occasions. The boxes are cycled back into the closet.

(Also: Birthdays, Fantasy)

CHILDREN

Mom's grandchildren live out of town and can only see her a couple of times a year, barely enough visits for someone who's always loved being around kids. At one point you'd even thought of borrowing your friends' grandchildren for a visit with her. But one day, while on one of your walks around the neighborhood, she strikes up a conversation with a five-year-old who lives a couple of houses down the street, and since then the two of them have developed a special relationship. They spend time in the garden, counting petals on flowers and arguing over images they see in the clouds. Mom chats away, telling stories that don't make much sense to you, but her five-year-old companion is totally engrossed. The little one brings her toys and books that the two of them read together. You serve them cookies and ice cream and appreciate having a respite. The visits have an uplifting and invigorating effect on Mom, and her five-year-old friend's delighted with this undivided attention. She seems oblivious to Mom's problems and accepts her, confusion, garbled speech, and all.

When her young pal can't visit, you and Mom go on picnics at the neighborhood playground or to the children's department of the local library. You even take her to fast food places where she's able to focus on a toddler and ask the mother, in the sweetest tone of voice:

"Would you by any chance consider lending us that beautiful baby of yours?"

You both leave the proud mother beaming.

Children are often able to communicate on a different level, without hang-ups or prejudices. They can get past screwed-up conversations and into a realm of feelings and a deeper under-standing. A few nursing homes have the staff's children visit for the day, while others combine their facilities with day-care centers for young children. The resulting interaction has been very beneficial for both the elderly and children alike.

(Also: Attitude, Empathy, Games, Singing)

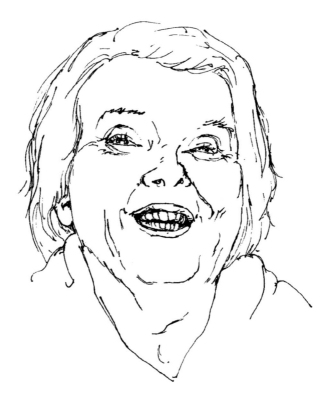

Some people make the world more special just by being in it.
-Anonymous

CHOICES

Mom's always been an independent and opinionated person. Now that you have to make decisions for her in most areas of her life, try to give her as much self-determination as possible by giving her choices as often as you can. Holding up two shirts, let her pick the one she wants to wear:

"How would you like to wear this blue-checkered shirt – or do you prefer this pink flowered one?"

At breakfast you give a choice of how she wants her eggs cooked and you try to be specific since she may not remember the terms herself:

"Would you like your eggs sunny side up or would you like them scrambled?"

If Mom has great difficulty expressing herself, you can phrase your choices so she can respond with a simple "yes" or "no."

"I promised you that we would go for drive today. We can go to the library or we can go to your favorite art gallery. How about the library?"

"No."

"Well, it sounds like you'd rather go to the gallery today. Is that right?"

"Yes."

Give only two choices at a time, making sure that you'd be able and willing to fulfill either of them.

(Also: Coaching, Communication, No!, Questions)

COACHING

Your wife looks at you in bewilderment. She has no idea how to get into the car. She needs your help, so you take her through the motions with gentle coaching. Approach this as though it's the first time she's ever gotten into a car. Guide her step-by-step in a clear voice, gesturing and demonstrating as much as possible.

"This is your seat (as you pat it.) First you step in here with this foot (as you pat her left leg,) then you sit down on the seat. I'll support you so you won't fall. Now pull your other foot in and move over to the middle of the seat. Perfect! There, you did it!"

You'll probably have to go through it all again the next time you go for a drive. With practice, your coaching will be as smooth as a flight attendant's safety spiel. Make sure that you are clear and precise, without sounding patronizing.

As you reach for a cup, your hand has already formed the shape it needs in order to grab it. You dash down a Manhattan sidewalk at rush hour and you don't stumble over the curb or bump into other people. As you go through the process of walking, your subconscious mind is constantly surveying and memorizing the terrain ahead. Any movement our bodies make involves this kind of subconscious planning.

If your husband is suffering from confusion, he may not be able to process his subconscious impressions. When he sees a fork, he may not remember what it is, so he's not able to prepare his hand to grab it. You can help him by placing the fork in his hand until he or his fingers remember what to do.

Your husband walks with hesitation and uncertainty because of his inability to plan ahead. You have become his "movement guide" as you describe out loud what is a few steps ahead, leading him gently by the arm.

You're coaching Mom through all sorts of everyday tasks, from how to use the toilet to how to button her blouse. You'll discover that your coaching will be easier if you alter your vocabulary and guidance. Mom's often confused about "left" and "right," so you can rephrase by saying "this one" and "the other."

"Are you ready to put on your shirt? Here, put one arm into this sleeve (as you hold it open for her) and then your other arm into the other sleeve."

"Come sit in this chair (as you pat the seat of the chair) and I'll sit in the other one."

"Here's your soup. This is the soup spoon. You can hold it in this hand" (as you place the spoon in her hand).

Mom may have forgotten the words for the parts of her body, so whenever you need her to do something specific, you can help her connect by patting her on her limb as you use the correct term.

"I'm going to turn on the water for your shower. Feel it with your hand (as you pat her right hand) and let me know if it feels comfortable to you."

Other directions may also baffle her, such as turning around or facing in a certain direction. If you say, "The glass is right behind you," she may have no idea what that means since she can't see it. Instead, go to her and gently turn her around so she can see it, guide her to a chair and place the glass in her hand while you offer her a reassuring remark:

"Here's your cup with your favorite juice. Come sit in this chair (as you pat it). Now you can enjoy your juice."

This step-by-step guidance may sound tedious, but it'll soon be second nature to you.

Dad doesn't want to brush his teeth. He may be reluctant because he's forgotten how to use toothpaste or may even have difficulty with the brushing itself. Try making a shared experience out of this task by brushing your own teeth at the same time. Chat about how he taught you to brush correctly, which will allow you to casually demonstrate for him:

"This is how you showed me when I was little. I still brush exactly the same way, see?"

If he can't handle the brushing himself, you'll have to do it for him. You're very sensitive to his feelings as you remind him of all the times he's helped you in the past:

"I remember when I had the mumps and you helped me brush my teeth. It was weird at first, but I was so glad to have clean teeth, thanks to you."

Explain everything while you're going through the process. Just to be on the safe side, have his teeth cleaned by the dental hygienist every three or four months.

(Also: Bathroom, Choices, Compliments, Eating, No!, Walking)

COMMUNICATION

"Mom, do you want to go for a walk?"

"NO!"

When you ask Mom "Do you want to take a walk?" she may not be sure at that moment what "walk" means. By saying "No!" to you, she won't have to make a decision about something that she doesn't understand, so she somehow retains her dignity and self-control. If your question is rephrased and preceded by a description or elaboration, she'll have more of a chance to process your question before responding.

Instead, present it in another way:

"Mom, it's so beautiful out. And it's springtime. Yesterday morning you made me promise that we'd go for a stroll around the block if the weather stayed warm. Maybe the daffodils will be in bloom in our neighbor's yard down the road. Come on, let's put on our walking shoes and go for a walk, okay?"

As much as possible, include Mom in the suggestion. Be positive and upbeat:

"I promised you this." (Meaning: this is something you wished for.)

Or: "This is your idea; I think it is a really good one."

Or: "You asked me to remind you that you wanted to do this now. I'm so glad I remembered."

Or: "This is one of your favorite things to do, isn't it?"

Avoid verbal traps:

"Do you want . . .?"
(unless you already know the answer, as in: "Do you want ice cream?")

Now that Mom has trouble expressing herself, you'll often have to speak and think out loud for her. Complete your sentences with "isn't it?" or "don't you think?" so she feels as if you're including her in the conversation:

"That was a good lunch, don't you think?"

Or: "I think this is good idea, don't you agree?"

Or: "Well, Mom, I was so bored with that movie, I almost fell asleep. I bet you couldn't stay awake either, could you?"

All Mom has to do is answer "yes" or "no," yet she feels as if you're asking for her opinion.

As you get used to this kind of communication, you'll find it much easier to deal with the more challenging situations.

"Friday's a good day for a bath, don't you think?"

Or: "I bet you need to go to the bathroom right about now, don't you?"

Or: "I'm tired and feel like going to bed, don't you?"

Or.   "Before you go home, Mom, I think we should have some lunch. I bet you'd like a sandwich, wouldn't you?"

(Also: Attitude, Choices, Empathy, Laurels, No!, Normal, Questions)

COMPLIMENTS

You're helping Mom get dressed. She has been kind of moody, so you find a detail to compliment her on:

"This shirt look so good on you. It brings out the color in your eyes."

"You look so pretty in your new haircut."

You have discovered that periodic sprinklings of compliments during the day help keep Mom from getting restless. When she starts to get agitated, you face her close and in a loving, intimate voice, you say:

"Have I told you lately, how happy I am that we are here together? I really enjoy being with you."

Or: "Mom, do you have a moment? I really need to talk to you. It always helps me to hear what you think."

And then you find some small "problem" she can help you with. From past experiences you probably know which of your "problems" is her favorite. It doesn't matter if you have used it many times before. If you think she might remember, you start with:

"I may have mentioned this to you this before, but ..."

You explain your "problem" to her in great detail with all seriousness and after she has given her opinion, which can be a simple "yes" or "no," you let her know how much you value her input and opinion.

"I'm so glad we talked about this. Discussing my problems with you always makes me feel so much better."

You keep a repertoire of compliments handy:

"You look just great in green."

"That haircut looks so good on you."

"You've always known what to do in this situation."

"Thank you for suggesting this."

"What would I do without you?"

"This is a wonderful idea. I'm glad you thought of it." (Even if it was your idea.)

"I'm so glad you taught me how to do this."

"You are the best: (gardener, cook, singer, or ...)."

" Will you help me with this, you're so good at it."
...and so on.

(Also: Affections, Dignity, Empathy, Laurels)

Nowadays we are all of us so hard up that the only pleasant things to pay are compliments.
                                        -Oscar Wilde

COMPREHENSION

Dad seems as if he's listening with rapt attention to your account of a trip to the post office until he says, with a big grin,

"All the balls are gone."

This response seems totally unrelated, but his facial expression suggests he thinks his remark suits your conversation. He has trouble expressing himself and there's no way of knowing how much he actually comprehends, but it's a good idea to assume that he understands everything being said by you and others, even if he doesn't give you an appropriate response. Include Dad in regular conversations, and always talk to him in a normal tone of voice. If other people are involved, you may have to be proactive and reiterate the conversation to him as you steer the others into talking directly to him, even if he doesn't respond. Conversations provide important stimulation for Dad. Whether or not he comprehends doesn't matter so much as the importance of being able to communicate his thoughts to the best of his ability.

☞

There are times when it's necessary that Dad really understands what you're saying: when you have to give him medication, get him into the bathtub, or buckle his seat belt, for example. In these kinds of situations, be calm while using a loving, normal voice. You may have to repeat your directions several times. If you start losing your patience, take a break and try again later.

(Also: Attitude, Communication, Empathy, Listening, Questions)

CONVERSATIONS

You're not sure how much Mom remembers. If you talk about something specific, you may put pressure on her to remember it. However, by talking in generalities, she has a choice of a "yes" or "no" or she may remember something that relates. Specifics don't really matter, as long as she feels the two of you are having a "conversation." You are not testing her memory, as long as you stay away from "Do you remember?" or put yourself in the same shoes by saying, "I don't remember, do you?" Then when she answers "No" you can share a chuckle over bad memories.

By using, "don't you think?," "weren't you?," "wouldn't you say?," you're keeping the channels open. She may start what sounds like rambling to your ear. Take a deep breath and listen to her with interest, as much as you can muster. She's trying to let you know that she's enjoying having a real exchange with you. It's the feeling that counts and not the contents. Keep your conversational tone on an adult level. Mom is not a child so don't speak to her as if she is one. Cutesy chitchat is demeaning to her and you.

Go with the Flow
You are listening to an "oldie" Glenn Miller tune, with Mom.

"What's the name of that? I don't remember, do you?"

"Harold."

"Oh, I thought it might have been "In the Mood."

"I got the book."

"Do you still have it?"

"I have to go home now."

"Gee Mom, we're having such a good time. Before you go anywhere, I'd like to share a bowl of strawberries with you. Isn't that a good idea?"

If you have the stamina and patience, you can go on like this for hours. Mom's delighted because you go with her flow and respond to her remarks, which makes her feel as if you're interested in what she says. You sprinkle your conversation with occasional compliments. When Mom says she wants to go home, you don't argue with her. Instead, you wisely divert her with strawberries.

Openers
"I may already have told you about this ...."

"I don't know if I told about you this, but ...."

"This happened a long time ago, so I don't know if you'd remember..."

"We met so many people and did so much today, it may be hard to remember ..."

Then you can proceed talking to her, as you would talk to a friend. She'll appreciate that you consider her an equal adult. As you're just relating thoughts, your own memories, or an interesting news event, you can go on chatting away as long as she seems interested. On the other hand, if it's important for her to understand you, slow down and enunciate clearly, repeating and rephrasing if necessary, always keeping your adult tone.

With Strangers

Mom got all dressed up to come with you to this party. People are talking to you and to each other, but Mom's not really able to participate because nobody says anything to her except for an occasional single-sentence greeting. It disturbs you that everyone ignores her, even though she's right there in their midst. Mom still enjoys being part of a group, though she might not be able to have a conversation in the usual sense of the word. There's no way of knowing how much she under-stands, but it doesn't really matter. It's likely she hears and perceives more than we assume.

People who are unfamiliar (and uncomfortable) with demen-tia may ignore Mom and talk exclusively to you, sometimes with inappropriate questions and remarks that can be disturb-ing or hurtful to her. An acquaintance asks you in front of Mom:

"So, she's the one with Alzheimer's, eh? Isn't she in a nurs-ing home yet? Gee, I can't imagine how you put up with . . ."

Interrupting your acquaintance is perfectly appropriate in light of her insensitivity. You stop her in mid-sentence by turning to Mom as you calmly rephrase the remark and make it clear that she has heard every inconsiderate word:

"Mom, as you can hear, this person's asking me about the tests you had done at the doctor's the other day, and she's ask-ing if you still live with me."

Turning to your acquaintance, you can add:

"We don't have the results yet, but you know what, it doesn't really matter, because Mom and I have a good time and we're so lucky we have this time together, aren't we, Mom?"

You must assume that Mom understood the insensitive comment so your interruption lets your acquaintance know that you consider Mom part of the conversation. Hopefully, you've made it clear that such callous remarks aren't very nice. If she persists, you'll want to be more direct and stand up for Mom by saying:

"Your remarks are thoughtless and unkind. Mom may have dementia, but she can still hear perfectly well. Would you please change the subject?"

ૐ

You and Mom are shopping at a department store, when a salesperson notices and comments about a bruise on Mom's arm. Mom's immediate reaction is to exclaim loudly:

"My daughter did that! She beats me and she locks me up. Hurry up, call the police!"

While the salesperson is trying to regain her composure, you grab Mom by the hand and head for your car. Safely at home, you have forgotten all about the incident until a police officer and someone from Adult Protective Services appear at your door. Yikes!

It takes a lot of phone calls and explanations to convince the two of them that Mom has Alzheimer's disease and the mark on her arm is a harmless bruise. They finally leave you with wishes of good luck.

You don't ever want to go through that again, so what should you do? You can understand why the salesperson had acted the way she did; after all, Mom looks normal and can sound totally lucid. The next time it happens, don't leave without an explanation. Having Mom wear a medical alert bracelet engraved with "Alzheimer's" will instantly convey her condition to others. You can also give Mom's bio and picture sheet to your local law enforcement agency and any emergency rooms in your area. If this happens again, ask the salesperson to call the police department to confirm Mom's situation so that you'll avoid all the stressful follow-up events.

(Also: Aggression, Baby Talk, Comprehension, Dignity, Identification, Neighborhood Flyer, Normal, Safe Return, Wandering)

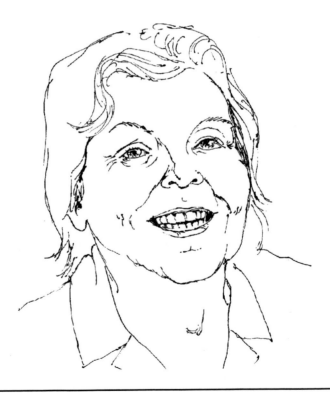

Conversation ... is the art of never appearing a bore, of knowing how to say everything interestingly, to entrain with no matter what, to be charming with nothing at all.

                -Guy de Maupassant

COUNSELING

Since Mom's been living with you, you've become extraordinarily patient and quite adept at holding back your feelings. Mom has become very responsive, and you're having a good time most of the time, but you've also paid a heavy price. It seems as if everything's always about Mom: her needs and her comfort while your own feelings get pushed to the side. You know that Mom's doing the best she can so you feel guilty for wanting your own needs met too. There are times when you find you're so frustrated that you feel as if you can't take another day. When these kinds of feelings well up in you, the feelings of guilt can also arise, making you feel even more stressed.

Try to share these feelings with your family or your Alzheimer's Association support group as often as you can. However, sometimes it's difficult to be totally free with the group. If you find that you're unable to open up, consider professional counseling for yourself.

A counselor or therapist can provide you with a truly safe place in which to vent your anger and resentment. Ask your friends for a recommendation or if that's not comfortable, talk to your doctor about a referral. Your local hospital may have a special group that you can join. Seeking counseling doesn't mean you're crazy, but repressing your feelings is. You need to let them out, look at them, and get some help looking for solutions. A therapist can be your best ally.

Your feelings are natural and seeking support is the healthiest thing you can do for yourself. If you're unsure about counseling, consider it something you can do that will help Mom as well as you. Her moods and behavior reflect yours. If you feel good, then she's calm and cooperative, but if you're upset, she can become more confused and cranky. If you can find relief somewhere, it will make life easier on both of you.

(Also: Anger, Forgiveness, Guilt, Home Help, Respite, Support Groups)

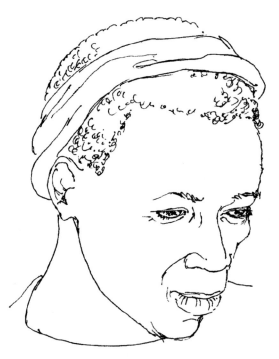

The more we care for ourselves, it becomes possible to care far more profoundly about other people. The more alert and sensitive we are to our own needs, the more loving and generous we can be toward others.

-Eda LeShan

CROWDS

You and Mom are browsing around her favorite department store. It's the big sale of the season so it's crowded and noisy. Hunting for the best sales was always the highlight of Mom's shopping excursions, so you are surprised when she becomes quite upset and pulls away from you. You can barely catch up with her as she makes a beeline toward the exit. You steer her instead to the shoe department, which used to keep her engrossed for hours.

"Mom, let's look over here. Maybe we'll find some new walking shoes. Look at those nice brown ones."

When you turn to her for the enthusiastic reaction you're expecting, she looks at you with tears welling up in her eyes. There's no choice but to quickly spirit her out of there. You hold her by the hand and gently talk to her about finding a peaceful little place to have a nice cool glass of lemonade.

Mom's probably suffering from sensory overload: too much noise, too many people, and too much going on all at once. Malls and large stores can be bewildering for someone who has trouble sorting out impressions, so consider shopping at smaller stores and boutiques.

The hardest situations for Mom are those involving relatives and friends who love her. She may feel overwhelmed and react with agitation at a large family gathering. Try to explain to everyone that Mom is easily unsettled by crowds and prefers one-on-one encounters. You can help her find a quiet corner and steer others to visit with her there.

(Also: Attitude, Empathy, Outings, Restaurants)

CURSING

Dad's been in his own world all afternoon. You've tried diverting him, but he just keeps pacing up and down the hallway. He's mumbling to himself when he suddenly lets out a loud tirade of curses, words you never heard from him before. Over the years he'd let out a "damn" and "hell" when he had a mishap, but he'd always apologize profusely to anyone within earshot. He once even washed your mouth out with soap when you were experimenting with creative language at age ten. Now he's exploding with a full repertoire of $*@'s and you are stunned. Your first inclination is to firmly stop him:

"Dad! What are you saying!? I don't allow that kind of talk in my house. Stop it right now!"

Instead, take a deep breath and try not to react. Remember that it's not uncommon for someone with dementia to display behavior that has been suppressed since childhood. Understand that Dad may not be able to control his actions. Relax and try to make light of it by joining him in a couple of expletives:

"$*#%* sure is a funny sounding word, when you really listen to it, isn't it?"

Try humor. Ask him seriously,

"Do you mean a big *&%@ or just a middlin' *$?"

Put his favorite comedy video in the VCR.

"Why don't you join me in watching this $#& show? It's really $&*# funny."

If you use his swear words in a normal conversation, he may hear that they're not so special and he'll become uninterested. Or you may choose to ignore them completely. It will have to be trial and error. If this occurs in public, gently say to him:

"Dad, this gentleman is not familiar with that word. Maybe you can think of another word."

Turn to the stranger and let him know what's going on:

"This is a phase of Alzheimer's. Please don't take it seriously."

(Also: Communication, Humor, Laughter)

If you can't make it better, you can laugh at it.
-Erma Bombeck

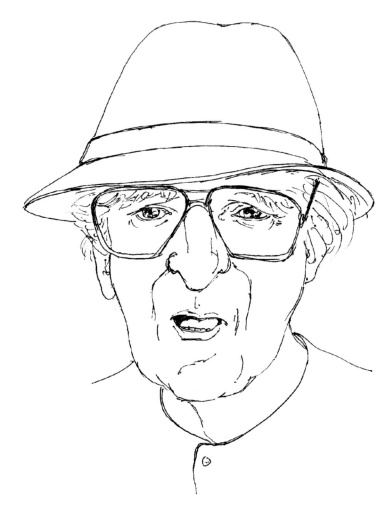

Develop interest in life as you see it; in people, things, literature, music -- the world is so rich, simply throbbing with rich treasures, beautiful souls and interesting people. Forget yourself.

-Henry Miller

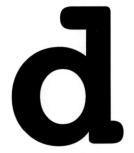

DAY CARE

You've always enjoyed your full time job. And now that Dad's living with you, you realize that you value it even more because it helps you stay grounded and connected to the outside world. By going to work and interacting with fellow employees or customers, you're experiencing stimulation, personal connection, and emotional support that creates a healthy balance in your own life. When you return home to Dad, you're more likely to feel renewed and recharged.

Dad used to be fine at home on his own, but lately that seems to have changed. He's withdrawn and sometimes depressed by the time you get back from work. When you ask him what he's had for lunch, he's so vague that you suspect he hasn't eaten a thing. You realize that he can't be left alone anymore and you need help looking after him while you're at work.

Some of the options open to you are home care, adult day care, or a senior center. At this point, adult day care seems to be the ideal solution, because it offers Dad both social interaction and mental stimulation. Because it's too difficult for Dad to enter-tain himself now and he's too forgetful to take care of his own meals, adult day care would remedy both these concerns.

When you return from work at the end of your workday, share an amusing or exciting anecdote from your day. If you had a dull day, make something up or retell an old favorite incident of his. Take the time to describe the smallest details with enthusiasm. Dad may not be able to give you feedback, but continue as long as he appears to be interested. He will appre-ciate that you consider him important enough to want to share your life experiences with him.

☺

Fortunately there is a growing awareness of the need for stim-ulating and safe day care for adults with special needs. Contact your state's Agency on Aging or the Ombudsman's Office for some suggestions.

(Also: Home Help, Respite, Share Care, Support Groups)

*The most effective way to cope with change
is to help create it.*

-L.W. Lynett

DEATH AND DYING

Many mourners are gathered in silence around the casket at the gravesite of an old and dear friend of Dad's. More are still making their way across the grass. You and Dad have been standing there for a while, when he loudly asks,

"When's the train coming?"

Heads turn and you are embarrassed. This is such a somber group, mostly strangers who aren't aware of Dad's dementia. You must admit that the crowd does look like a bunch of commuters waiting for the 5:24 Express. You quietly explain to him that this is not a train platform but rather a funeral for his friend John. He seems to accept your explanation and watches the late arrivals in silence for a while. Surveying the crowd, he says,

"No wonder John's not here. He's such a happy person and everyone here's so sad."

You decide that Dad doesn't really grasp what's happening and doesn't need to be exposed to any more sadness, so you lead him back to the car. Stuck in the lineup of parked cars, you take the opportunity to talk to Dad about his own wishes.

"This has been an awfully serious service. It sounds to me as if you think John would have liked something different. When I go, I want everyone to have a wonderful time. How about your celebration? What would you like?"

Dad flashes a big grin.

"I want happy music, good food, chocolate ice cream, and lots of good stories."

Although you've always known it was inevitable, the thought of Dad's dying has always depressed you. The two of you have never talked about it until now, yet under these circumstances it seems so easy.

"I promise we'll have a great party for you. But I have to tell you, Dad, that I'll still be sad, because I'll miss you very much. However, we don't have to worry about it for a long time, thank goodness. As soon as we can get out of here, let's go test ice creams, okay?"

You fill the rest of your wait in the car talking about the trees and flowers around you and other unrelated topics. Dad has completely forgotten why he's there. You contemplate your conversation and make a silent vow to yourself to try to make each day with Dad a day worth remembering.

You've spent the last months or years making a wonderful life for Mom. You've shared joys and laughter with her and you've filled her life with many special experiences. In recent times, she's become quite weak and withdrawn. You suspect that the end might be near. You're hoping that she'll go quietly in her sleep, just as she always wanted.

Yet the final episode may include having to take her to the hospital. If she's terminally ill and there's nothing more that medicine can do for her, then you have two options: to let her life wind down naturally or to keep her on life support indefinitely. You have her Living Will in place that states her last wishes. If she does not wish to have life support once she has reached this terminal stage, then you need to decide if you want her to die in a hospital or at home where you can keep her comfortable in her own bed and in her own surroundings.

A social worker at the hospital can put you in touch with hospice or personnel who can help with her care at home.

Keep her environment and routines as normal as possible. Even if she's comatose, you can still read to her or talk to her while playing soothing music in the background. This would be easy to do at home, but at the hospital you'll need to bring a small cassette or CD player with head phones so she can listen to her favorite music. It's recognized that the awareness of music is the last sensation to go. The music will drown out hospital noises and help create a peaceful environment.

Whether Mom's at home or in the hospital, talk to her in your normal, gentle voice. If she's at all aware, she needs to hear that you're there with her. She also needs to feel your touch; so hold her hand as much as possible and give her a gentle back rub or foot massage. It might be difficult for you, but try not to let your own fears and sadness show through. Mom may be aware of her own impending death, so let her know that you're aware as well. One approach might be:

"Mom, I love you and I'll miss you a lot, but it's okay for you to leave any time you wish. We're okay and we can take care of everything."

If she's able to talk, she may need to express her fears and anxieties. As good as you are at communicating with her, this will be the toughest test for you yet. You need to be Mom's pillar of strength at a time when you yourself are devastated.

If she's comatose, hold her hand or rub her arms. Then you might gently say to her:

"I love you, Mom. Everything's been taken care of. It's all right for you to rest now."

And if she's religious, you can add,

"The angels are waiting for you, Mom. God loves you and I love you."

ॐ

Tip! Final arrangements are much easier to deal with ahead of time. Confer with several mortuaries about costs and arrangements, so you won't be forced to make decisions while you are in an emotional state. You've already talked to Mom about her last wishes, especially regarding cremation. Ask her doctor to instruct you on procedures you can expect at the time of her death.

(Also: Affection, Dignity, Empathy, Massage, Normal, Paperwork)

There are two ways to spread light; to be the candle or the mirror that reflects it.

-Edith Wharton

DEMENTIA

Mom was the one person in the family who kept track of everyone's birthday and anniversary, calling the rest of you to remind you to send a card or a bouquet of flowers. Mom used to be so sure of herself, outgoing, and quick to break into a smile. Lately things have been so different. This woman, who was known as an impeccable dresser, sometimes is dressed in inappropriate outfits and has even shown up disheveled at family gatherings. She is becoming withdrawn and anxious and will break into tears at the smallest upset. Mom, who was the keeper of the family archives, has trouble remembering the names of her own children and sometimes even denies furiously that she has any grandchildren.

You fear that she may be developing Alzheimer's disease. But before you jump to the conclusion that she has Alzheimer's, keep in mind that many people develop dementia from disorders that may be reversible.

It's important to distinguish between normal "senior moments" like forgetting your grandchild's name and more seriously forgetting that you have a family. Periodic memory lapses are normal. Our brains will retain and regurgitate facts quickly as long as there's a natural connection to something else current in a thought train. In other words, it's harder for any of us to remember something completely unrelated or out of the blue. As we get older our brains have so much more to sort through to recollect a specific thought.

Mom's memory lapses may be ordinary "senior moments." But if she is increasingly confused and you detect drastic changes in her personality, such as agitation, anxiety, or depression, you definitely will want to have her condition checked out. She may be in the early stages of Alzheimer's disease or she may be suffering from a reversible type of dementia. There are dozens of causes of dementia aside from Alzheimer's, including malnutrition, vitamin deficiencies, dehydration, allergies, drug reaction, anemia, depression, or adult-onset diabetes, which could be causing her dementia. Many of these are correctable.

If Mom's dementia has come on suddenly, you'll want her to see her doctor immediately. Bring with you a complete list of her food and drug intake, including prescriptions, over-the-counter medications, vitamins, and alternative supplements. Mom should have thorough physical examinations, including MRIs and CAT scans, which are particularly good for detecting brain tumors, fluid on the brain, and blood clots. Request extensive blood tests and discuss tests for possible food allergies.

(Also: Alzheimer's Disease, Alternative Remedies, Diet, Vitamins)

It's such an act of optimism to get through a day and enjoy it and laugh and do all that without thinking about death. What spirit human beings have.

-Gilda Radner

DEPRESSION

Mom will sometimes burst into tears without any obvious provocation. She may be suffering from depression. It may stem from her feeling useless and out of place. You can talk until you're blue in the face about how much you love her and want her to live with you, but it won't help until Mom regains some sort of self-respect and feels like a contributor again. Let her know that you need her help. Be sincere, because if you gush too much, all your good intentions could backfire and she'll feel ridiculed and further alienated.

Using our suggestions as a guideline, design a few activities specifically tailored to Mom's interests. Start slowly with a small project and build it up as she responds. Your first projects should help her to feel useful. Ask her honestly for her opinions and suggestions and always listen patiently to her reply, even if you don't really understand it.

If you have tried every approach outlined in this book and she still doesn't respond, it may be time to seek professional help for her. There are antidepressant drugs available by prescription, but they may have serious side effects. Read the circulars for specific drugs before making a choice. An alternative is St. John's Wort, an over-the-counter herbal remedy that has shown excellent results as an antidepressant. Make sure you confer with a health professional and keep a journal of Mom's emotional state, her activities, and her responses. As she improves, talk to her doctor about reducing or discontinuing the antidepressant medications.

(Also: Activities, Alternative Remedies, Diversions, Humor, Laughter, Personal Space, Projects)

DIET

Regardless of the cause of Mom's dementia, you can help her enormously by making some changes in her diet. You will want to eliminate foods high in saturated fats and sugar, both of which aggravate dementia. Next, talk to her doctor about putting her on a strong multivitamin with minerals and adding vitamin E and ginkgo biloba.

Alzheimer's is a deterioration of nerve cells in the brain. Although we do not have a cure yet, there are things you can do that may help slow the progression or at least improve Mom's health in general. A low-fat and low-cholesterol diet is a very important start.

❧

Leafy vegetables, red onions, fresh citrus fruit, and even coffee are high in bioflavonoids, antioxidants that support the work that vitamin C does. Recently bioflavonoids have been found to lower cholesterol as well.

Carrots, squash, sweet potatoes, and cantaloupe. Pink grapefruit, and tomatoes. Any fruits or vegetables with an orange or red hue are good sources of beta-carotene. Beta-carotene converts into vitamin A, which is essential for cell growth and development. Dark green leafy vegetables also provide beta-carotene.

Canola oil, flaxseed oil, walnuts, fatty fish (sardines, herring, swordfish, and salmon.) Polyunsaturated fats, also known as Omega-3 fatty acids, prevent heart disease and fight cancer.

Soybeans, tofu and soymilk, lentils, chickpeas, and kidney beans are excellent sources of isoflavones, which provide estrogen-like compounds when estrogen is low, and they also provide protection against breast cancer.

Water Elderly folks in general are notoriously conservative in their liquid intake. Mom's generation considered water something you used to take your medication or to rinse after brushing your teeth. They must find the current preoccupation with designer waters puzzling. Keeping that in mind, if Mom resists drinking plain water, you can create refreshing and healthy "ades." Mix frozen juice with twice the water suggested on the can and add sweetener to taste. The goal is eight glasses a day. Alcohol beyond a single drink a day. Excessive alcohol use has been linked to the development of Alzheimer's disease.

(Also: Alternative Remedies, Alzheimer's Disease, Vitamins)

Be careful about reading health books.
You might die of a misprint.
                    -Mark Twain

DIGNITY

You and Mom are having a lovely lunch at your favorite restaurant when suddenly she has a funny, distracted look on her face. You ask her if she likes the food and she mumbles that it's really good, so that's not the reason for her expression. You ask her if she needs the toilet, but she shakes her head. Then you happen to notice the tag of her tea bag hanging out the side of her mouth. You reach across the table and gently remove the tea bag with a napkin. She's already bitten into it and her mouth is full of loose tea, so you say to her:

"That doesn't taste very good, does it? Go ahead and spit it out in this napkin and then you can rinse out your mouth with some water."

The folks sitting at the table next to yours have witnessed this and are staring, but you ignore them and continue to help Mom spit the tealeaves out into the water glass and ask the waiter for a fresh glass of water. This has never happened before and you're a little shaken, but by treating this as if it's a perfectly normal occurrence, you help Mom maintain her dignity and good spirits. After she rinses her mouth she quickly forgets about the whole incident and continues her meal. You can consider the possibility of finding an alternative to restaurant dining if her growing confusion continues to cause such awkward moments.

It can be a task at times to maintain Mom's dignity, but with your positive attitude and relaxed approach, you'll manage to get through these moments by reminding yourself that no one has ever died from embarrassment.

Mom needs you to be the guardian of her self-respect and dignity, especially as her confusion increases. You speak out on her behalf in ways you never would have imagined. It took a while to build up your nerve, but now you interrupt others who insist on using patronizing baby talk to her and you stop people who speak about Mom as if she wasn't there. Mom may not be able to let you know in words how much she appreciates your interventions on her behalf, but her behavior will tell you.

(Also: Affections, Attitude, Body Language, Compliments, Laurels)

I care not what others think of what I do, but I care very much about what I think of what I do. That is character!

-Teddy Roosevelt

DISCUSSIONS

Mom has always been intrigued by science, history, and anything else based in fact. You watch PBS with her and read to her from Scientific American, The Nature Journal, and National Geographic Magazine. Though she's not really able to discuss much with you, she never takes her eyes off you whenever you read to her. Even when you read the same thing for the tenth time, try to approach it as if it were the first time and read it with the enthusiasm and gusto of discovery:

"Listen to this, Mom. I found a really provocative article. I can't wait to share it with you. I bet you'll like it, I found it very interesting. Would you like to hear it right now?"

Since you've read it to her before, there's a chance that she'll interact with you so you can stimulate a discussion by sharing ideas with her:

"Do you recall when we were in school that we learned the dinosaurs had become extinct but we didn't know why? Well, in this article they suggest that dinosaurs became extinct within a couple of years after an asteroid crashed on earth by the Yucatan Peninsula. Hmm . . . interesting, don't you think? They also say in this article that the skies throughout the world would have been so darkened with dust as to block out all sunlight. Wow! Yeah, I guess that would destroy an awful lot of vegetation in no time at all, huh? And there wouldn't be anything for the dinosaurs to eat, so of course they'd become extinct. Gives you something to think about, doesn't it?"

Serious adult discussions are as important to Dad as they are to you, even if he's not able to contribute much anymore. Think about what you talk about with your friends and try to discuss the same with him. You can talk about a subject you know he's interested in or consult with him about something happening in your personal life.

"Dad, I could really use your advice on something important to me. I'm considering moving my office at work. Tell me what you think, okay? My office now has a good view but very cramped space. I can move into a bigger space but it doesn't have a view. What would be important to you: more space or a better view? Oh, and another consideration: the smaller office with the view is close to the bathroom and the other one is close to the water cooler. What would you do?"

Give him enough time to react in between your questions. If he responds with a totally unrelated remark, go with his flow, no matter where it goes. You may have to slow down and simplify your choice of words but talk to him like an adult and avoid using a condescending tone. Engaging in adult conversations helps Dad maintain his self-esteem and dignity, even if his responses are incoherent or disjointed.

(Also: Communication, Conversations, Listening, Normal, Questions)

The most wasted of days is that on which one has not laughed.
-Nicolas-Sebastion Chamfort

DIVERSIONS

Aunt Elsie has been living with you for the last couple of years. Every so often she'll become obsessed with wanting to "go home." She's standing at the front door in her overcoat, with a pair of bedroom slippers in her hand. She announces "I'm going home now!" and she starts to turn the door handle. You quickly go to her side and put your arm around her shoulder as you say,

"Okay. I'm so sorry you have to leave so soon, Auntie, because we were having such a good visit. Oh, I almost forgot something. I promised to show you those new earrings I just bought. Come, let me show you."

Aunt Elsie loves jewelry, so she gladly follows as you retrieve your jewelry box. You sit her down at the kitchen table with the box in front of her as you slip off her coat:

"Let me take that, it's too hot in here for a coat, isn't it? I'll hang it up in the closet for you. And let's set your slippers in the closet by your coat, then you'll know where they are, okay?"

She looks at the earrings and before long she's settled in with the entire contents of your jewelry box laid out on the kitchen table, arranging earrings in matching pairs. As you talk with her about some of the pieces, she becomes so totally engrossed in all the glitter in front of her that she's forgotten all about wanting to leave. You haven't argued with her about wanting to go home; instead you've diverted her attention. You changed her mind by changing her environment, and you also ended up sharing some special time with her as well.

Your husband is restless and irritated. He's started pacing and mumbling angrily to himself. You've tried offering him tea, to no avail. You leave the room and come back with today's mail as you say:

"Darling, I'm really busy right now. I sure could use your help. Would you mind opening the mail?"

You hand him a blunt letter opener. He cheerfully starts opening the mail, so you add:

" . . .and while you're at it, would you mind sorting it? It would be great if you'd put all the bills in one stack and the rest in another stack."

You might find this such a successful diversion that you can encourage it as a daily activity.

(Also: Activities, Compliments, Normal, Personal Space, Projects, Reality)

Happiness is not the absence of conflict, but the ability to cope with it.
                                        -Anonymous

DRESSING

By Oneself

Mom wants to continue to dress herself for as long as she is able, though you'll want to keep an eye on her to make sure she's dressing somewhat appropriately. She may need some assistance with which is the front or back of a dress, or which shoe is right or left. She may have trouble with "left and right" so use "this one" and "the other" instead.

"This shoe goes on this foot (as you pat her leg). Now you put the other one on the other foot. There you are, ready to walk!"

If Mom still selects her own wardrobe, she may forget that she wore that same outfit yesterday. Maybe she chose it because it's hanging right there in the front of the closet or maybe it's because it's her favorite dress. To discourage her from picking the same clothes all the time, go to her closet when she's not in her room and remove the often worn outfit so that it's not available in the morning for her to wear. If that doesn't work, the next time she reaches for that same old dress, distract her by offering her another one.

"How about this blue dress, Mom? You look so pretty in blue. It makes your eyes shine."

@

The two of you have been invited to lunch at a friend's house and Mom has been in her room getting dressed. After forty-five minutes you decide to check on her. She is beaming as she says:

"I'm almost ready!"

She's wearing three skirts on top of her slacks, along with two scarves. First take a deep breath, then say,

"Wow, that certainly is a creative outfit you've got on. But, you know what, it's kind of hot today. I think you'll roast in all of those clothes. How about choosing just one outfit? I like the skirt with the flowers. It goes so well with your blouse. Let me help you."

Getting dressed can be a confusing experience. Panties have three openings and Mom may not be able to discern into which opening to place her foot. A dress can also be a nightmare and it's easy for Mom to get tangled in a full skirt. She may need a guiding hand from you. When you help her, keep it dignified and talk about how you experience similar problems with your own clothes.

Buy Mom attractive garments that are comfortable, non-binding, and one size larger. Have Mom wear socks instead of stockings, and buy loose fitting queen-size knee-high nylons that won't cut off her circulation, in case she attends an event where wearing hosiery is absolutely necessary.

Use undershirts instead of brassieres. Mom may find a turtleneck uncomfortable; instead choose a boat neck, crew neck, or cowl neck. If she often undresses in public, clothe her in outfits that button or zip in the back. Bring extra clothes with you in the car: a change of pants, a sweater, a top, and extra pads.

Makeup
You help Mom with bathing and brushing her teeth. You comb her hair and watch her discreetly as she gets dressed. She has always worn makeup and still tries to apply her own lipstick,

at times with interesting results. Her favorite color is bright red, which she shakily applies to chin and cheeks as well as lips. Looking at herself in the mirror, she seems satisfied with her appearance and you've learned to live with it.

This is not a problem at home, but when you go out in public, Mom often draws startled glances from strangers. You're good at ignoring the puzzled looks, but one day at church, the stares are so obvious that Mom becomes confused and uncomfortable.

The next day the two of you visit your local department store makeup counter. You distract Mom by having her browse through scarves and handbags while you have a quick conference with the sales person. When Mom eventually sits for her "make over," the sales person makes a big point of using a nearly colorless lip-gloss, touting it as the latest in fashion while complimenting Mom on how beautiful she looks with the new color! Discard her fire engine red when you get home. Mom can now apply the lip gloss anywhere she wants with no visible trace. You may have to wear colorless lip-gloss yourself in Mom's presence and reserve your red lipsticks for evenings out.

Shaving
Dad used a straight razor all his life with great macho pride, but there's no way he can use one safely now. You've tried to convince him that wearing a beard is very manly, but even you have to admit he looks kind of shaggy. Every time you've suggested a regular razor, he protests and besides, you're worried that he could still hurt himself. You can solicit help from a male friend of his or yours to talk to him about how mascu-

line "new" electric razors are. At first he may be reluctant, but the friend can probably convince him that it's completely manly. Now he can shave himself for hours on end, sometimes driving you crazy with the noise, but it's worth it considering his clean look and the fact that he hasn't lopped off any ears yet.

(Also: Coaching, Compliments, Dignity, Resources, Undressing)

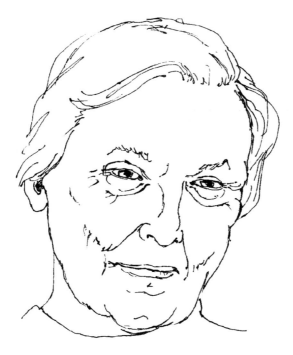

The greatest thing a human being ever does in this world is to see something .... To see clearly is poetry, prophecy, and religion, all in one.

-John Ruskin

DRIVING

Dad's still driving, though not quite like the old days when he practically lived in his car. Usually he does well, but lately he's been missing a lot of turns and has trouble reading road signs.

Recently he was driving the two of you down the freeway when he missed your turnoff. Without thinking you exclaimed,

"Oh Dad, that was our exit! You missed it!"

He stopped the car cold, switched into reverse and backed up, oblivious to the rest of the oncoming freeway traffic.

Home never looked so good to you before. You stumbled up the front steps on your Jell-O knees, thanking every deity you could think of and pledging to them all that this was the last time Dad would ever drive again!

Boy, that is easier said than done! This man loves his automobile with a passion. It's his pride and joy, and a symbol of his freedom. Losing his car will break his heart. You've tried to discuss the subject with Dad before and your otherwise gentle father hits the roof and wants to hear nothing more about it.

Since the freeway incident you've made up all kinds of excuses for why he should let you drive. You've tried to take his keys away, and you've even disconnected the battery. These actions kept him from driving, but Dad's becoming obsessed with his car and is suspicious when you tell him the car isn't working. He grumbles angrily,

"You just don't know anything about cars and that mechanic of yours doesn't know what he's doing."

Dad's best friend offers to help. While you tell him about the incident on the freeway, Dad emphatically states that he would never do anything of the sort. You know that there's no point in arguing, so you take a deep breath and say instead,

"Dad, you are a very good driver, but I'm worried about you when you have trouble reading the signs. I love you and I wouldn't want anything to happen to you."

This calms him down and Dad's friend suggests a gradual tapering off. Reluctantly Dad agrees that he'll only drive the two of you on your weekly visits to his sister, using a side street route he "knows" like the back of his hand, and to a couple of shops that are just around the corner.

You promise not to overreact as you did on the freeway and that from now on you'll gently guide him to the next turn without sounding too much like a back seat driver:

"Let us take the next turn. That'll get us to the right street."

You want to help him stay focused and calm. You won't mention missed turns. That would only aggravate him and most likely make his driving even scarier.

When the time comes, you can ask his doctor to give Dad an official "medical order" requiring him to give up the car keys. Contact your local Alzheimer's Association for advice and guidance if you anticipate difficulties. You'll also want to encourage Dad to talk to others, who have had to give up driving, so he doesn't feel so alone. Your local senior center may also be a good source.

Car Safety

You've been driving along with Mom, when she grabs the door handle and cheerfully announces,

"Well, I'm going home now."

Of course she's wearing her seat belt and you always lock the car door, but it still shakes you up. Try to stay calm as you say:

"Mom, please wait until the car has stopped."

Mom may not always be aware that she's in a moving vehicle, even while sitting right next to you, the driver. You keep chatting away, talking about the driving itself to remind her that she's in a car. If she's fidgety, you talk to her about how she's feeling. She may not be able to tell you that she's too hot, too cold, or too uncomfortable, so her first instinct may be to get out of the car. Reassure her by letting her know that you're aware of how she feels:

"I know you're tired of being in the car, Mom. We're going to be there soon and then we'll get out. We can stand it a little longer, I hope."

And when you reach your destination,

"Phew, that sure was a long drive. I'm glad we finally made it, aren't you?"

Tip: Keep an emergency pack in your car. Also consider having an extra outfit, a sweater, and a couple of pads or half briefs on hand if you're to be away from the house for longer periods.

(Also: Coaching, Communication, Emergency Pack, Empathy, Listening)

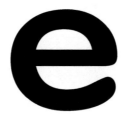

EATING

Mealtime is the highlight of Dad's day. He carefully tucks his napkin in at his throat or at least he makes a good attempt at it. His mother was a stickler about manners. Most of the time meals go well, but there are times when he appears confused. He'll stare at his plate and the utensils, apparently uncertain of how to get the food into his mouth. You place the fork in his hand and close his fingers around it.

"Dad, this is your favorite. It looks good, doesn't it? Here, you can use this fork to eat it."

You get into a habit of having only one utensil available at a time, which seems to help. You precut his food into bite-size pieces and arrange them on his plate to look appetizing.

His beverage sometimes confuses him. He may try to "eat" it with his fork or pour it over his dinner. You gently take it out of his hand, as you say,

"I'd be glad to hold your drink for you while you eat, okay?"

You fix him a fresh plate and keep the drink separate, or hold his fork while he takes a sip.

You make sure that you don't mix foods needing different approaches on his plate. Only fork food or only finger food, like potato chips. If his hands have forgotten how to hold a sandwich, you can cut it up to become fork food. If you're eating at a restaurant, ask to have the contents of the sandwich served on a plate as separate items.

There may come a time when handling a utensil becomes too confusing for Dad. At that point you can change his diet to finger food. This may be a challenge, but can also be interesting for you to create a well-rounded meal of finger food, such as steamed chunks of vegetables, pieces of chicken, and fruit.

@

You used to be amazed at Mom's self-control. She'd eat so little at dinner you wondered why you missed out on those thin genes. Now that she's living with you, however, you're growing concerned that she's getting too thin. She takes tiny little bites and chews each one forever.

Whenever you're finished with your own meal, you'd routinely ask her,

"Are you finished with your dinner?"

To which she'd always answer, "Yes."

Then one night you by chance you phrase your question differently and ask instead:

"Mom, are you still eating your dinner?" to which she responds with a "Yes."

It takes her forever to finish what's on her plate. An hour later, you finally clear the table. It dawns on you that she's probably always been a very slow eater and in the past she would just automatically stop eating as soon as everyone else did, even if she was still hungry.

Now you routinely ask her: "Are you still eating?" rather than "Have you finished?" and you allot enough time for her to eat. She's putting some weight back on her bones, which makes the extra time worthwhile.

(Also: Body Language, Choices, Coaching)

It's difficult to think anything but pleasant thoughts while eating a homegrown tomato.
-Lewis Grizzard

EMERGENCY PACK

You'll want to carry an "emergency" pack with you in the car:

• A standard first aid kit.

• Important papers.

• Phone numbers, including doctors' and emergency numbers.

• Extra clothing: sweater, pants, and underpants.

• Several panty liners or half briefs and an under pad.

• Tissues, packaged wet towels, lotion, and sunscreen.

• Entertainment and diversions: a favorite book or magazine, a word game book, a songbook, a joke book, peppermints, or hard candies.

In winter: extra scarves, gloves, leggings.

(Also: Incontinence, Paper work)

Look at everything as if you were seeing it either for the first or last time. Then your time on earth will be filled with glory.
-Betty Smith

EMPATHY

You'll be more effective in handling Mom's problem situations if you can empathize with her by looking at circumstances through her eyes. Learn to share her reality, even when it's very different from yours. How would it feel to be in her shoes?

What does her dementia feel like to her? Picture yourself frantically searching for your car keys, but you can't remember where you left them. Now imagine that you've finally found them, only to discover that you have absolutely no idea what you're supposed to do with them or even what they are.

Can you imagine what it would feel like to experience that sort of confusion every single day? In your own mind you are the same person you've always been. You still think of yourself as normal, but the world around you seems to be changing. You try to explain your dilemma to a familiar-looking person, but the words just don't come out right. You feel as if you're going crazy and you start to panic. The familiar person looks at you with gentle eyes and says, "May I have a hug, please, Mom?" You let her hold you as calmness washes over you. You even giggle. Maybe you're not losing your mind after all. Slowly that familiar-looking person becomes recognizable: it's your daughter!

Other people, however, are starting to treat you strangely. One person pats you on the head as if you're a dog while another coos in your face as if you're a baby. People are starting to ignore you, and even worse, they talk through you as if you weren't even there. Your feelings haven't changed; you still feel joy, pain, longings, and love. Doesn't anybody see?

As Mom loses her ability to communicate, it might feel to her as if she were a stranger in a foreign country, completely ignorant of the local language and customs. She tries to explain that she needs help, but as hard as she tries, no one seems to understand.

You're learning to be empathetic with Mom and look at the world from her point of view. It helps you gain an understanding of her feelings, but there are still times when she catches you off guard.

You're surprised to find Mom dissolving into tears. You have no idea why. When you ask, she utters forlornly:

"They left without me."

"Who left without you and where are they going, Mom?"

"They're going to the service. My sister could've waited for me. How could she do that to me?"

You comfort her while you review your family history to recall any event that could have triggered such a reaction. Then it hits you! Mom's reliving her beloved grandmother's death, when she had been left at home during the funeral. You need to find a way to soothe this heartbroken ten-year-old child.

"I'm so sorry that they didn't take you, Mom. I didn't get to go either. Come with me and we'll light a candle for Granny."

When you "go into the space" with her, your empathy helps you understand and share her feelings so that you can deal more effectively with all kinds of situations.

(Also: Attitude, Coaching, Comprehension, Diversions, Normal, Reality)

ENVIRONMENT

Dad's toy car has been with him since he was six years old, though it has little paint left after so many years of handling. As a matter of fact, you even played with it when you were small. It now sits between the portraits of his parents and your baby picture. You carefully dust around them because he has a fit if he thinks they've been moved. They're all in perfect view from his favorite old easy chair, which, like the toy car, is an antique of indeterminable age and indistinguishable color. You've tried in vain to convince him that he needs a replacement.

As Dad gets more confused, his environment becomes increasingly important to him. As tempting as it is to give a fresh new look to his room or apartment, you resist the urge. If you have to move him into another space or room, try to duplicate his former room. He needs the comfort of his favorite chair being in its usual spot in front of the chest on which all the family pictures are positioned in their familiar places. If you must make changes, do so gradually. Introduce his new recliner in place of the old monstrosity by keeping a throw blanket on the old one for a few weeks, then transferring the blanket onto the new recliner, which you position in exactly the same location as the old one.

(Also: Privacy, Signs, Transitions)

Happy times and bygone days are never lost ...
In truth, they grow more wonderful within the
heart that keeps them.

-Kahlil Gibran

EXERCISE

We often hear it said that exercise is critical to mental and physical wellbeing. Dad needs to move his body. Try to get him to raise his arms above his head and swing them back and forth. Unless he's wheelchair bound, have him walk with you with as much vigor as he can safely handle. You can also make up your own versions of exercises for Dad. How about taking him for a barefoot walk on the lawn in the back yard or on the shoreline of the beach? Throw your arms up to the sky and make noises, oinks, moos, caws, and hollers. Challenge him to a lion-roaring contest. It's a wonderful feeling to let it all out and it happens to be good exercise for Dad. You might want to borrow a child or two to help you out. Most of us adults are a little self-conscious and need practice to feel free and loose again.

Dancing

If Mom's somewhat agile and mobile, you can reintroduce her to the fine art of dancing. It's been a while since Mom last danced, so you start slowly, watching her balance and avoiding turns or spins. Stay in one spot on the dance floor and move your arms and upper body to the music. When Mom joins in, you simply synchronize your movements to hers. If she's reluctant, grasp her hands lightly and move them to the music. It may take her a while to get back into the swing of it if she hasn't danced in a long time. Keep it light and spontaneous as you improvise your dance movements to her favorite music, whether she loves Puccini, Tommy Dorsey, or Garth Brooks.

You're playing one of Mom's favorite operas, Madama Butterfly. The music never fails to inspire her. She smiles and her eyes begin to shine as she starts swaying to the music. You move your chair so that you're facing her wheelchair and begin moving your arms in concert with hers. At first you're both a little shy about your movements, but soon you're both doing ballet with your upper bodies. It's so much fun that by the time the music stops you're both breathless but probably laughing at the sheer joy you have shared.

If Mom has serious problems with her speech or if she is non-verbal, these movement explorations can give her a meaning-ful outlet for self-expression.

Sitting

Mom needs exercise but she doesn't move well enough to take walks anymore. Instead, the two of you can sit in straight-back chairs facing each other and do sitting exercises. Later on you and Mom can bring these exercises to your share care group, making them even more fun when they are shared with others.
See: Sittercises at the end of this segment.

Swimming

For years your favorite exercise has been swimming, so after Dad moved in with you, he'd join you at the local pool. He's a strong swimmer, or at least he was. Lately you've noticed moments of hesitation in the middle of his familiar strokes, as though his body is forgetting those very basic moves. Dad's not aware of these changes and when you point this out to him he gets quite upset. Before he has an episode that could endanger his life, introduce him to water aerobics, exercises that can be done in the shallow end of the pool. Dad should be wearing a swim vest that will keep him afloat.

Walks

Dad enjoys his walks around the block with you. If his eyesight is good enough, you can take the time to look at details along the way: a budding flower, a newly painted wall, or an ant colony. Later on you can recollect your adventures.

"It sure is a beautiful day today and we had a great walk. We walked all around the block this afternoon. I really enjoyed it, and you did too, didn't you?"

"Yes."

"We were looking at those beautiful flowers growing in front of the neighbor's house. We couldn't think of the name of them and you thought we should go the nursery to see if they can tell us. We can go later this week, if you like. Does that sound good?"

(Also: Body Language, Coaching, Communication, Crowds, Music, Walking)

Happy people plan actions, they don't plan results.
-Dennis Wholey

Sittercises

Do the following exercises 3 to 5 times each. Use gentle movements with a slow and deliberate pace. Avoid jerky movements and skip an exercise if Mom complains about pain.

Raise arms, breathe in. Lower arms, exhale.

Extend arms out front, palms up, then down.

Reach down side of legs to touch toes.

Bend chin to chest, then look up at ceiling.

Raise shoulders up to ears.

Lean forward, then pull back to row. Sing "Row, Row Your Boat."

Raise arms, breathe in. Lower arms, exhale.

Extend one arm to opposite shoulder.

Extend other arm to opposite shoulder.

Stretch one leg up slowly, then the other.

Stretch one arm to ceiling, then the other.

Keep heels on floor. Tap toes.

Keep toes on floor. Tap heels.

Raise arms, breathe in. Lower arms, exhale.

Extend arms out front, make fists, then open.

"Punch" one arm out front, then the other.

Stretch arms out front, bend wrists down, then bend up.

Stretch arms out front, circle wrists.

Shake out arms.

Extend both legs, point toes out, then up.

Raise one knee up to chest, then the other.

Raise arms, breathe in. Lower arms, exhale.

Clasp hands together, circle as if stirring a big pot.

Clasp hands, raise above head, then down in front, as if chopping.

Raise arms up, touch head, shoulders, knees, toes.

Roll shoulders.

Raise arms, breathe in. Lower arms, exhale.

Give yourselves a big hug.

We need 4 hugs a day for survival.
We need 8 hugs a day for maintenance.
We need 12 hugs a day for growth.
- Virginia Satir

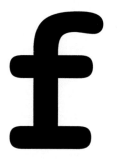

FAMILY

You're hosting a large family gathering, the first since the start of Dad's decline. The family is coming from out of town and hasn't seen Dad in quite a while. Call everyone before their arrival to give them a clear picture of Dad's current state. Carefully explain how to communicate with him: avoid using the phrase "Do you remember?" Discourage the use of baby talk, and refrain from talking about him within earshot.

So what happens? Dad is sweet and positively lucid, at least at certain moments. Somehow he instinctively knows to keep quiet enough to cover up his confusion. He even responds to the dreaded "Do you remember?" question with an innocuously firm, "That sure was something!"

At this point, you suspect your siblings are probably convinced you're grossly exaggerating Dad's condition. You try to tell your brother that Dad's behavior today is unusual, but your brother's response is patent skepticism.

Through it all, Dad's having a wonderful time and thanks to his flawless behavior, the family is still completely ignorant of the challenging experiences you confront while caring for him. However, you take advantage of the situation: while everyone's feeling so positive about Dad, you ask your siblings to share in the caregiving in order to give you a break. You persist until you get commitments from each of them for specific dates when Dad will be staying with them.

There is no way your family can empathize with you unless they can acquaint themselves with your experiences. If they live out of town and Dad can't travel, invite them to stay at your place where they can look after Dad. When they do, take advantage of the respite by actually going away someplace. You know that if you stick around, you'll continue to be responsible for the work involved. A few days will barely give your sibling a taste of your daily life, but on the positive side, the experience might give him or her a chance to bond with Dad. It isn't that you're trying to prove anything to your siblings so much as you just need to make it clear to them that you need and deserve their help, support, and understanding. The caregiving of your father is a family responsibility, so be insistent that they participate.

(Also: Communication, Crowds, Respite, Visitors)

Ignorance gives one a large range of probabilities.
-George Eliot

FANTASY

Your afternoon plans have been ruined by a sudden downpour. You're both disappointed, so you try a fantasy trip instead:

"Gee. Look at that rain, Dad. It's too bad; we had such great plans. Our trip to the rose garden will just have to wait for a sunny day. Now, I have a suggestion: how about flying to Paris for dinner at Maxim's?"

Dad looks puzzled, but you continue without missing a beat:

"We can spend the night at an exclusive hide-away on the Isle of Capri. Then we'll fly to Cairo for breakfast and tour the pyramids before lunch. Do you think we should bring a picnic or should we zip off to Kenya for a safari?"

Dad's still not giving you a reaction, so you decide elaborate to get a little more fantastic:

"Nah, I think we should climb to the top of one of the pyramids and take a rocket to Mars. I've always wanted to see the red sky of Mars. How about you? I wonder what kinds of food they serve in Martian restaurants. "

At this point he probably grins, having caught on to the silliness of your fantasy, so you continue,

"We could take the first morning flight out and finish up by going to the opera in Sydney, Australia."

"I don't like opera."

"Okay, then we can go to Kyoto, Japan instead. You've always liked Japanese food and you love Japanese gardens."

You can continue this fantasy game indefinitely. Ask Dad where he'd like to go next and elaborate on each location. If you're not familiar with it, make up something fantastic and ask for his suggestions or corrections.

◎

Dad has wonderful memories of family picnics when he was a child. All through your childhood you'd heard the stories about these legendary events, though he can't really talk about them lucidly anymore. Now, whenever you want him to feel really special, you'll suggest planning a picnic just like the old days:

"D'you know, it's supposed to be beautiful weather on Sunday. That's what the weather reporter said on the news. How about a picnic in the park? We could go to the deli and get a picnic lunch like your mother used to make. I still remember that special sausage she'd always buy. It was some sort of salami, wasn't it? And then we'll finish up with a luscious, gooey brownie."

You can spend a whole evening planning your picnic, right down to the very last detail. Food is one of best topics for day dreaming together and in the process you can recall favorite childhood memories.

(Also: Activities, Future, Humor, Laughter, Outings, Projects)

You see things and say why?
But I dream things that never were; and I say Why not?
-George Bernard Shaw

FIXATIONS

All of a sudden Mom won't eat if there's more than one item on her plate, or she separates the mixed vegetables into little piles which get cold by the time she starts to eat. After a few weeks of this, you adjust your cooking and serving to suit her new habits. Serve one food item at a time during a meal. Or consider serving her meat one day, then vegetables the next while making sure her total intake of food is balanced and nutritious.

You're out for a stroll, holding Mom by the arm, when you realize she's not looking where she's going. She's focused on fingering the buttons on her blouse. You get her attention for a minute or so, but then she's back to fussing with the buttons. She succeeds in undoing a couple of them. This new behavior persists whenever she wears a blouse with buttons. Your simple solution is to change to pullover tops and back-buttoned tops.

Dad manages to find the tiniest specks. He finds them, real or imaginary, on the car seat, on your friend's jacket, on the windowsill, and on his plate. He laboriously picks them up and holds them in his fingers. If you try to convince him that he can let them go, he gets upset and insists on holding them. He may finally relinquish them if you present him with a container specially labeled "SPECKS."

(Also: Diversions, Signs)

Presence is more than just being there.
-Malcolm S. Forbes

FORGIVENESS

Your sister has been a thorn in your side for a long time now. Ever since Mom came to live with you, she's been criticizing your every decision and action. She won't come to see for herself what's going on, but in her mind there's nothing you can do right. You're fed up with the hostility she evokes in you. Whenever the phone rings on Saturday mornings, you get a sinking feeling in your stomach and the anger rises in your throat as you realize it's her weekly telephone call.

So far you have had sole responsibility for Mom, so you know you don't have to put up with this kind of harassment. Yet you feel guilty about your negative reactions because, after all, she is your sister and you're supposed to love each other. You've tried to tell her that her attitude hurts you, but she doesn't seem to listen. She makes you angry and unhappy, so now it's time for you to take a stand and tell her that you don't want anymore negative phone calls. Write your sister a note and let her know your new resolution: positive phone calls or no telephone calls at all. Insist that she takes her turn caring for Mom and maybe she'll realize that her judgments of you have been too harsh.

When you are confronted with these feelings, give yourself ten or fifteen minutes to acknowledge your anger, wallow in it, and then let it go, while you forgive yourself for just being human. If it continues to bother you, then talk to your counselor or therapist about it.

Things happened between you and Dad when you were a kid that still trigger unresolved anger and hurt in you. Now Dad is living with you because he has dementia but he has absolutely no recollection of those events from long ago. As much as you've tried to stifle it, the rage still sometimes wells up inside you and it makes living with Dad very difficult. You've heard about the importance of forgiveness, but Dad's dementia makes it impossible to talk to him about this.

Forgiving him without a confrontation and acknowledgment on his part is virtually impossible for you. How do you deal with it when the perpetrator has grown old and demented? Confronting him with the truth at this point may give you some relief, though it may disturb Dad so much that he retreats even further and becomes either deeply depressed or overtly angry and agitated, which will make your life with him even more difficult. Is it worth it? You may decide that Dad is a different person now and try to accept him as he is. You can forgive yourself for feeling anger or rage at the Dad you used to know.

There are times when outrage is appropriate, as in the case of physical abuse, molestation, and violence. Recognize that your feelings about what happened are real, and what Dad did was unforgivable. Your rage is justified. With the help of a counselor you may be able to make peace in your heart with your past, even if Dad isn't acknowledging any of it. You need to find release from this pain and you deserve to be set free in order to grow and move on.

(See: Counseling, Guilt, Support Groups)

Forgiveness does not change the past, but it does enlarge the future.
-Paul Boese

FRIENDS

Dad's fortunate enough to have an old friend living nearby. You've made arrangements with the friend's caregiver so he and Dad can spend time together at least once a month. His friend's about as confused as Dad, but the two of them still have the best time when they get together to reminisce about old times. By now you're quite used to hearing the same old stories repeated again and again whenever the two of them are together and you've come to realize that the stories themselves aren't important; they're a way to express the love he and Dad share. As you sit back and watch, you see them as they are to each other: a couple of high school kids. This is a priceless time for both of them and you feel privileged to be able to share it with Dad. If you have access to a video camera, this is a good time to use it.

@

Mom came to live with you from her home in another state. You realize that she needs friends of her own, but her social skills are pretty much gone, so she relies on you for her total companionship. Your share-care group's been good for her, because she's become friends with one of the women. Neither of them remembers the other's name, but it doesn't seem to matter. The two of them greet each other as long-lost friends whenever they meet. You and the other caregivers help them out with their conversations; otherwise they'd probably remain silent throughout the whole visit. During lulls in the conversation, you may be uncomfortable with the silence, but you notice that they seem totally content just being there with each other.

(Also: Communication, Conversations)

FUTURE

"Dad, I thought we'd go to the library tomorrow. Then after lunch, we can take a drive down along the river. How does that sound?"

Dad's big on making plans. When you were a kid the family's summer vacation was already planned long before the daffodils even began to bloom. Now he relishes discussing the next day's doings, which may be real or fanciful, because by morning he may have forgotten most of them. Should he remember something that doesn't fit in with your plans, you can redirect him with an enthusiastic alternative:

"I have a surprise for you. The other day you wanted to go to the library (or the store) but it was closed. Well, we can go today. How about that? That's good news, isn't it?"

Making plans is synonymous with "the future." We all need to feel we have some sort of future, although in reality we know nothing is ever a certainty for any of us. "Planning" what you'd like to do in the future can be a cheerful experience. Just think of the times you've fantasized about winning the lottery!

"You know, Dad, I've been thinking we should take a visit to that little hideaway you like so much. There's that neat bookstore and cafe where we can read some good books and eat lunch. They make great turkey sandwiches with avocados and sprouts. Then later we'll drive around the corner to the ice cream parlor and have a big scoop of ice cream in a sugar cone. What flavor would you like? Chocolate with almonds? Kiwi fruit with macadamia nuts? Or Guinness stout ice cream with beer nuts?"

You make it up as you go along, making sure to include Dad's favorite things. His responses will tell you where to go next. The point is that you're not making a promise; you're merely painting possibilities for the future.

(Also: Empathy, Fantasy)

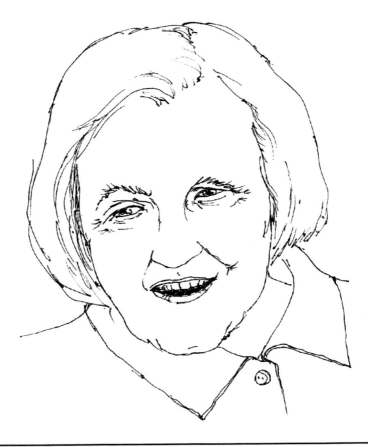

The secret of health for both mind and body is not to mourn for the past, not to worry about the future, or not to anticipate troubles, but to live in the present moment wisely and earnestly.
–Buddha

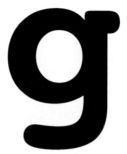

GAMES

Bingo, bridge, canasta, jacks, tiddlywinks, horseshoes, ring toss, badminton, Ping-Pong, pin the tail on the donkey. . .

Dad may not be able to play many of these games anymore, but you can create simplified and noncompetitive versions of ones that he might really enjoy. Perhaps he liked playing bridge, so you can make up a new "game" vaguely reminiscent of bridge: deal each of you a few cards and then take turns laying down the cards according to suits. The purpose of the game can be how quickly you both can lay them out. He may also be able to play a game of solitaire, as long as you play it with him.

He might be able to play open-handed poker: draw five cards from the pile, lay them face up on the table. Together you can decide which cards to keep and which ones to discard or replace. You can keep going until you have a decent poker hand, no matter how long it might take to get a good one.

There's nothing wrong with games of competition as long as Dad's having fun. If you notice that he's becoming frustrated or agitated, change to a noncompetitive, non-skills game, or simply take a break and do something else for a while.

@

Mental stimulation continues to be extremely important for Mom. Encourage her to participate in conversations and ask for her thoughts and ideas. If she enjoys crossword puzzles and other word games, look for game books in the magazine section of your supermarket. You'll find books for varying abilities, so you can select the appropriate level. Mom needs to be challenged but not overwhelmed.

When she reaches a point when even simple crossword puzzles and other word games are too difficult for her to do on her own, Mom can "help" you instead.

Outdoor Games
Outdoor games can be anything from ball toss to croquet. Beach balls are easy to toss and soft and gentle to catch. Go to a local toy store and buy a variety of balls in different sizes (preferably Nerf foam balls). Many children's lawn games won't feel juvenile as long as you take them seriously. Consider ring toss, horseshoes, or lawn bowling. Be sure to shop for the plastic, nonlethal versions of these games.

(Also: Activities, Fantasy, Projects, Personal Space, Word Games)

GARDENING

Your childhood home was surrounded by vegetable gardens, herb patches, and flowerbeds, all tended lovingly by your mother. After you and your siblings grew up and moved out, your parents were transferred to the city and your mother started a full-time job, so she had to be content with a couple of window boxes hanging off her apartment balcony.

Mom's living with you now. You take her on outings, you cook together, and once in while you get a chance to read with her, but there are long periods of time when you're distracted with your own work and Mom is left to her own devices. She goes out of her way not to disturb you when you're working and she spends most of her time wandering around the house. You've tried to set up an "office" for her but she's not interested, so you don't know what else you can do. Then one morning you ask her where she'd like to go for the day's outing and she says, "The nursery, it's time for spring planting." Aha! You had forgotten about her passion for horticulture.

Start with a single flower box. Encourage Mom as she selects seedlings, plant food, gloves, potting soil, trowel, and watering can. Before long she is tending two more flower boxes, which makes getting around the apartment a bit tricky, but the maneuvering is worth it just to see the joy on Mom's face.

If you're lucky enough to have a yard, you can set up a small area for Mom to plant a vegetable or flower garden. Later you can enjoy the fruits of your labors later with a special dinner, whether it's vegetables or a bouquet of flowers.

(Also: Activities, Kitchen, Outings, Projects, Personal Space)

GOING HOME

Every so often Mom will stand at the front door with a load of clothes in her arms. With great determination she announces:

"I'm going home! I have to leave now. Just leave me alone! I don't want any favors from anybody. I don't want any rides or anything like that. So I'm going to walk and it's twenty miles, so I have to leave right now!"

You've tried reasoning with her, reminding her that she sold her condo and moved across country to live with you, but she gets very angry, accusing you of lying to her and keeping her prisoner. Sometimes she'll announce:

"I have to go home now. My mother's waiting for me and she'll get very angry if I'm not on time."

It becomes clear to you that there's something else going on. It's not simply a matter of returning to her own condo; she's talking about her childhood now. You put your arm around her and say,

"Your mother called and said she'll come over here later. She insisted we should go ahead and eat dinner now."

On the other hand, Mom may still be aware on some level that her mother's no longer alive. In that case, be very gentle with her as you explain,

"Mom, your mother's been gone for several years now but it's still so hard for me to believe. Sometimes I pick up the phone to call her before I remember that she's no longer with us. But I'm so glad that you're living here with me now. Before I forget, we need to go to the store because we're about to run out of chocolate ice cream, and that would be a catastrophe, wouldn't it? Let's go right now, since you already have your coat on."

This kind of scene could be an indication that Mom is feeling insecure, lonely, or without purpose. Getting her involved in her personal space would be good diversion:

"You were telling me earlier about a new painting you've started. I'd really like to see it before you go."

Or you can start a project that the two of you can enjoy doing together. It could be something that she used to enjoy like sewing, gardening, or cooking.

"Before you go, Mom, would you please help me with the salad dressing. I love that special recipe of yours and I just don't have the hang of it yet."

You don't argue with her about her wanting to leave, you simply suggest a postponement to her. With a good distraction, she'll soon have forgotten about her intentions.

Your diversion should be a project so it's short and manageable in order to give Mom a sense of accomplishment. She may be painfully slow now, stretching your patience since you end up doing most of the work, but you'll succeed in making her feel useful and involved. When the project is finished, give her a good hug and a sincere compliment.

"I'm sure glad you're helping me with this. It would have taken me forever to do this without you. Thank you so much."

(Also: Affections, Compliments, Diversions, Reality, Personal Space)

GUILT

You're doing so well with Dad that your friends have nominated you for sainthood. Most of the time this is great to hear, but there are other times when heavy feelings of guilt envelop you because you know you could do so much more. Your relationship with Dad is becoming more and more lopsided as you constantly give while Dad constantly takes. You're aware that the circumstances make this inevitable, but as your situation becomes more extreme, you may question your own feelings and actions. We're used to getting strokes or feedback from the people affected by our good deeds. Dad's not able to give you positive reactions anymore, so the reassurance you might need to let you know that you're doing the right things is replaced by doubt and guilt.

You can't help but feel burdened with this task you've taken on and may find yourself envious and resentful of your siblings or friends who are free to pursue their own lives. If you're trying to juggle Dad's caregiving with a full-time job while taking care of your own family, then you definitely have a full plate. You may get a lot of help from your family, but you still feel it's your responsibility, and there are times when you're overwhelmed with guilt for inevitably neglecting one or the other.

You're being only human to blame Dad and his condition for your situation and there may be times when you wish he'd die so it would all be over. It's very hard for us to talk about these "dark" thoughts or to even admit to ourselves that we harbor them. We have all felt them at one time or another, so forgive yourself for being normal. The next time Dad drives you to the edge, take a deep breath and find a diversion for him, so you can retreat to the most peaceful place in your house and have a good cry. Or give yourself a good hug and promise yourself to take some real time off in the very near future. Tomorrow night get a sitter for Dad and go to a movie or dinner with friends. Look into respite care that will give you some time for yourself on a more regular basis.

As Dad's condition deteriorates, you know that it's only a matter of time before you'll no longer be able to care for him at home. You've started looking into care facilities in your area, but it's with a heavy heart because you feel the weight of guilt and a sense of failure. You know that it's important for Dad to have what's best for him, and as hard as it is to admit, which might ultimately be a care facility. Your rational self knows there is no reason for you to feel guilty. After all, you've given him a home for a long time now, and you know that even if he moved into a care facility, you would still be there for him.

Your feelings and thoughts are normal. Try to share them with your Alzheimer's Association support group, even if it may be very hard to talk about them. Start by discussing the weakest negative feelings and then work your way up to the really scary ones. Everyone in the group will most likely share your feelings of guilt over very similar thoughts. If these subjects have not yet been dealt with, the group will probably be relieved that the subject has finally been broached. You are involved in a tremendous undertaking so you're entitled to dark thoughts and doubts like any other normal human being. Our culture disapproves of negative thoughts and we've been scolded since childhood for expressing them, so when they pop up, they automatically trigger our guilt reflexes.

If you feel overwhelmed and these feelings are so frequent that they interfere with your personal wellbeing and your effectiveness as a caregiver, then talk to your family about one of them taking over the caregiving for a while. At the very least, ask one of them to stay at your house for a couple of weeks or longer so you can take a vacation. You may feel selfish to want time for yourself and this can lead to additional guilt feelings. However, needing a break doesn't mean that you're letting Dad down or that you've failed. A break gives you a chance to think about your situation and realize that you've undertaken the most difficult task of your life and that on the whole, you're doing a fine job of it.

(Also: Care Facilities, Counseling, Respite, Support Groups)

Holding on to your anger is like grasping a hot coal with the intent of throwing it at someone else; you are the one getting hurt.

-Buddha

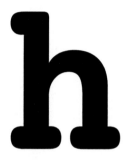

HALLUCINATIONS

Dad is a war veteran. No one really knows what kinds of nightmarish experiences he underwent while in combat. He'd always refuse to discuss what happened, shrugging it off with a "What's done is done." However, in his dementia, some of those old fears are coming back to haunt him. He fixates on an enemy he thinks is coming to get him:

"They know where I am. They're coming. Oh, what am I going to do?"

You have no idea who "they" might be, but it doesn't matter; what he needs is comfort and reassurance that he won't be harmed by anyone.

"You're safe here, Dad. I'll never let them hurt you. Besides, they don't know this address and we have a good strong lock on the door. Would you like to see it?"

You may have to make some "phone calls" to "authorities," once you find out which ones he'd trust. Within his earshot, but with the phone disconnected, say:

"Hello, is this the FBI? I'm double-checking our security arrangements. Will you please confirm that they don't know our address? . . . Thank you so much. I feel so much better now."

Then you can say,

"Yes, Dad, the FBI agent just told me that your file is secure and they are making sure that nobody knows of your where-abouts except the people we want to visit us or call us. The FBI agent also said we can call him anytime we have a con-cern. He was awfully nice and helpful. You don't have any-thing to worry about. You are perfectly safe here with me."

@

You're having lunch with Mom, when she suddenly exclaims,

"Get that bear out of here!"

You start to protest that there's nothing there, but you stop yourself. Take a deep breath as you get up and say to her,

"I bet he's hungry. I'll take him outside and feed him."

Go through the motions of taking the "bear" out of the room, closing the door behind you. When you return, be serious when you say,

"It's a good thing you told me. He was really hungry, so I gave him something to eat and now he's gone back to the woods. Are you ready for some more iced tea?"

Mom's hallucinations are totally real to her. To help her come back to reality, you can "go into the space" with her to help her remedy the situation, and then you'll be able to divert her. "Going into the space" with her means that you join her in her experience, with empathy and sensitivity. When you're able to feel what she's feeling, you're more likely to be successful in bringing her back to the present.

(Also: Diversions, Empathy, Honesty, Loving Lies, Reality)

Patience and fortitude conquer all things.
-Ralph Waldo Emerson

HOARDING

One day while you're are cleaning Mom's room, you find two bars of soap stashed under the bed. Several days later you discover two more bars in the top drawer of her bureau. No wonder you're running out of soap in the bathroom! You explain to Mom that the soap is supposed to be kept in the bathroom. She nods impatiently because of course she knows that bar soap belongs in the bathroom, but it's likely that she'll forget what you've just told her ten minutes from now.

Mom is a child of the Depression and has always been a fanatic about saving things, even tiny slivers of soap, so you decide to try a different approach. You get a basket, put a sign on it saying "Soap" and put it on her chest of drawers. Fill it with the slivers of soap from her various hiding places. After a few weeks, you can suggest that she keep the basket of soap in the bathroom instead. Buy liquid soap for use in the bathroom, since you know she doesn't understand how to use it and she'll likely leave it alone.

If this doesn't work, or if she's hoarding a variety of different items, consider installing childproof locks on all the cabinets and drawers so you can lock up anything that you don't want Mom to hoard. Continue checking her room frequently for stashes, but it wouldn't hurt to leave a few of her favorites in place. You'll also want to check all garbage cans and wastebaskets for stashes, just in case she has decided to hide her glasses or dentures there.

(Also: Home Safety, Signs)

HOME HELP

You've decided you need help looking after Dad. Until now, you've been doing everything by yourself: all the cleaning, cooking, and caring for Dad. Your energy is used up by the routine maintenance, leaving you with little time or energy left over for any pleasure and stimulation for both of you. Here are some possible options on home help:

Family

Your first conversation should be with your siblings and other family members. Work out a respite schedule where someone stays with Dad for a week or two at a time or have him stay at their homes for a change. Be very insistent with them; this is the kind of situation where everyone must pitch in. Caring for Dad should be a responsibility that is shared by all of you.

If you have family living nearby, ask any of them to help every so often by cleaning your house or cooking a meal. This will free you up to do something more enjoyable with Dad.

Housekeeper

You can hire a full-time housekeeper to help with daily household chores and upkeep, or consider a part-time person to come in once or twice a week to do the laundry and the floors. This person will most likely be interacting with Dad, so make sure that you share some of this book to help them in their communication with him.

Personal-Care Aide

If Dad is having problems with physically getting around, you can hire a personal-care aide to come in daily or even just a few times a week in order to help Dad with his baths, shaving, or other physical situations that you may need help with. You can check with your local agency of aging for referrals to qualified agencies or individuals. Any time you hire a private aide, you'll want to check references and qualifications.

Personal Companion

If you're working full time, you might consider hiring a companion for him. This person can give Dad intellectual stimulation by spending time with him in your home, and by reading, discussing, or playing games with him. A companion can take him out on picnics, to the library or museum, and to other places he enjoys. You might want to check with a college nearby to see if there are any students interested in a job. It's important of course that Dad enjoys the company of his companion and that they're compatible. Besides checking applicants' references, you'll want to make sure they're open to new ideas and approaches in caring for a person with Alzheimer's. Observe as your potential assistant interacts with your Dad. Does he treat Dad respectfully? Do they seem to enjoy each other's company? Under your supervision, Dad's new companion should have a few trial runs using the approaches outlined in this book so that he understands how you expect your Dad to be treated.

(Also: Day Care, Family, Respite, Share Care, Support Groups)

Just do what you do best.
-Red Auerbach

HOME SAFETY

There are several safety measures you can take without having to remodel your entire house. It is worth hiring a professional to install shut-off valves for the water and concealed switches for electrical hazards. The kitchen and bathroom are primary trouble spots, but don't forget about garages and storage sheds.

Windows and Doors

Your front door should have a lock that Mom cannot open by herself, like a double deadbolt, and place a stop sign or a sign on the door that reads: "Do not go out this door." You can position similar signs on any other doors that you want to keep secure. If that fails to work, try hanging a curtain in front of the door or install a full-length mirror on it.

If you live in an upper-level apartment, make sure all your windows are secured and have appropriate screens. If you have a balcony, secure the door, but go ahead and use the balcony with Mom whenever weather permits.

If you live in a rural area and Dad is prone to wandering, you'll need to have your yard is securely fenced with locks on the gates and make sure that Dad always wears an identification bracelet.

Kitchen

If Mom likes to fiddle around in the kitchen but you're worried about accidents, you can take precautions by making a few safety changes:

Kitchen checklist:
- Keep sharp knives out of reach.
- Use childproof closures for any cabinets that you want to secure.
- Keep all household cleaning stuff out of reach.
- Keep small appliances unplugged or off the counters.
- Remove the knobs from the stove.
- Remove stopper from sink.
- Unplug garbage disposal and dishwasher.

Bathroom

You'll want to install grab bars in the tub or shower and place a large safety mat in the bottom, if the tub or shower doesn't already have a nonskid bottom. You can either install a grab bar by the toilet or use a safety rail.

If your husband routinely turns on the water and leaves it running, you can avoid flooding by removing the stoppers in all your sinks and tubs and install a "ball valve" water shutoff under the sink. As an added safety measure, turn your water heater thermostat down to a tolerable temperature to prevent him from scalding himself.

Bath times will be much easier and less contentious if you use a hand held shower in place of the stationary showerhead. When you first turn it on and lead Dad into the shower, let it hang down. It's less frightening that way.

Transfer all medication out of the medicine cabinet and into a cabinet that is inaccessible to Dad. You'll also want to keep all household cleaning solutions out of reach. It's easy for Dad to confuse mouthwash with dishwashing liquid, especially if they both have a lemony smell.

Bathroom checklist:
- Install grab bars in the tub or shower.
- Place a large safety mat on the floor of the tub or shower.
- Install a safety rail beside the toilet, with a booster seat.
- Replace your showerhead with a hand held shower.
- Keep all household cleaning chemicals out of the way.
- Put all medications in an out-of-reach or locked cabinet.

Tip! If Mom has trouble finding or using the toilet paper holder, get a standing paper towel holder, set it on the counter or on the floor next to the toilet, and use it for toilet tissue. It's bigger and easier to see. Keep an old-fashioned bar of soap at the sink. Liquid soap is a newish invention and she may not understand how to use it.

Fire Safety
Review your house for anything that can cause accidents. Mom means well, but she doesn't always remember what she's been doing. She may have turned on the stove with the intention of making you a cup of coffee and then forgotten all about it. You want to keep matches and lighters out of her reach if they represent a temptation to her. It's lovely to have dinner by candlelight, but make sure you don't leave the candles unattended. Buy a couple of fire extinguishers and place them in strategic spots, like the kitchen and near the living room. Have them inspected annually by the fire department.

(Also: Identification, Neighborhood Flyer, Signs, Safe Return, Wandering)

Acceptance of what happened is the first step to overcoming the consequence of any misfortune.
-William James

HONESTY

Dad is still cognizant of many events in his life and you're usually able to discuss them honestly with him whenever he brings them up. Your mother died quite a few years ago and Dad remembers that fact most of the time. Yet there are other times when he slips into a long-ago reality as he anxiously waits for her to come home. Most of the time you're able to help him recall that she has died, but there are other times when he gets agitated and accuses you of lying. At those times when he cannot hear the truth, you may have to resort to telling a loving lie, even though your family has always been sticklers for honesty. It feels awkward at first, but you realize that there are moments when a slight untruth becomes the kindest response you can give to him. In order to be convincing, however, your loving lies should be realistic and based on a truth of some kind.

"Mom will be late. She wants us to go ahead and eat our dinner now. She doesn't know what time she'll be here."

If your mother was an intellectual, then use an answer that would have fitted in with her real interests:

"She had to stop at the library to do some research. She was always so serious about her research, wasn't she? How about us going to the library tomorrow? Or maybe the hardware store. What do you think?"

You've gently turned the conversation away from his concern about your mother and into something involving your relationship with Dad.

@

Mom has been diagnosed with Alzheimer's disease. You wonder if you should tell her the truth about the diagnosis. It's a tough decision. If she's already forgotten about the tests and the doctor's visit, then you'll probably just want to leave it alone for the time being. Nothing will change drastically in the near future, so try to relax and carry on as usual with your lives.

If Mom is still in the early stages of the disease and insists on knowing, then you'll just have to trust your instincts about what you tell her. Be aware that hearing she has Alzheimer's disease can be devastating for her. On the other hand, it can help her understand what's been happening to her lately. Keep in mind that science is not yet able to distinguish with certainty between different types of dementia and Alzheimer's disease. Discuss it with her, but follow up with reassurances that you'll be there and help her along the way.

"Mom, when we went to see the doctor today, she said you have dementia. That means that you forget things and sometimes you get confused. Well, you could have told her that, right?"

Give her a hug and continue with:

"I'm so glad you're living here with me so I can help you with the remembering."

Then change to another unrelated and more upbeat topic.

(Also: Alzheimer's Disease, Attitude, Empathy, Guilt, Loving Lies, Reality)

To understand is to forgive, even oneself.
-Alexander Chase

HOSPITAL
In-Patient

Mom has to spend time in the hospital. You've already made sure that the word "Alzheimer's" is clearly written on the front of her chart. She fell asleep last night without any trouble and you finally went home to get some rest yourself. You arrive this morning to find Mom wide eyed and on the verge of tears. She's struggling against restraints tied to her wrists and ankles. You feel dizzy with anguish for her and run to the nurses' station. What had happened to cause so drastic a measure? The head nurse, in a soothing (i.e., patronizing) voice explains:

"Your mother was quite unmanageable this morning. She refused to eat her breakfast and she screamed and struck out at the nurse who came to bathe her. We routinely restrain and sedate our Alzheimer's patients for their own safety. Everything will be fine. She doesn't understand anyway."

Your insides are churning and boiling. This is Mom, your sweet mother, trussed up like a Thanksgiving turkey. You know how reasonable Mom is in spite of her dementia. Didn't anyone even try to communicate with her? You're seething as you approach this supercilious nurse. Take not one, but two very deep breaths as you say:

"I will see to it that someone is here all day with my mother. While we're here your staff can bathe her and take care of other activities that may cause a problem. Let's do this without using restraints or sedatives."

You run a crash course for the staff on how to communicate with Mom and how to gain her confidence. Sharing this book may help. You'll want to stop anyone in their tracks if they start using baby talk. If Mom needs to undergo a procedure, ask the technician to explain it to her step by step, in a normal tone of voice, and repeat if necessary. If she resists bathing in these unfamiliar surroundings, ask the staff not to bathe her for a couple of days, then help the staff with the baths until she feels safe with them.

Hang a few of her favorite pictures on the wall that faces her bed. If there's no music or radio available, you can bring a small tape player from home and play music she loves. You'll want to stay with her as much as you can for the next few days, so arm yourself with a substantial collection of books, pictures, puzzles, and songs. Your intention is to have as much fun as possible, no matter how serious her condition is. Laughter is an amazing healing tool. Encourage her to participate as much as her physical condition allows. Sing together and "dance" to Mozart or Duke Ellington. This is guaranteed to look weird to anybody who peeks into her hospital room. That idea alone can bring you some good laughs:

"Those other people must think we are nuts, huh? Boy, they don't know how much fun they're missing, do they? I think we should invite them to join us, don't you?"

Mom's hospital stay will be the best you can make it. She'll heal much faster if she is surrounded by familiar things: food, pictures, music, and you. If she's not on a restricted diet, you can supplement the hospital menu with goodies from home. Whatever Mom's ailment is, you want to get her back home as fast as possible.

Mom has a broken hip. After surgery and a few days of obser-
vation in the hospital, she'd normally be sent to a rehabilita-
tion center for several weeks of physical therapy. Let her doctor know that you want to bring Mom home as soon as possible. Find out whether or not Medicare or Medicaid will pay
for a physical therapist to come to your home.

Many hospitals have case managers who will work with you
on "after care." They can help you organize a home-care solution and help you meet with social workers and/or occupa-
tional therapists in order to retrofit your home to suit Mom's
special needs.

Outpatient
Dad has to go to the hospital as an outpatient. To keep him
from getting unnecessarily anxious, wait until you're on the
way to the hospital before you explain to him what's going to
be happening. He'll take his cues from your attitude and
words. Stay calm and upbeat, but straightforward and honest
about what to expect and then reassure him that you'll be
there with him.

The hospital usually requires patients to arrive a couple of
hours ahead of time. You know Dad would go nuts waiting
that long, so you call the supervisor and tell her that Dad has
Alzheimer's, so you need the absolute latest appointment
time. You also ask her to double check to make sure that
"Alzheimer's" is written big and bold on the cover of his
chart. Amazingly, hospital personnel are often not prepared to
handle special situations like dementia and Alzheimer's.

You stay with Dad through all the prepping, explaining the procedures to him, maybe not correctly, but at least convincingly. If he is only going to have local anesthesia, you can stay with him throughout the procedure so you can help him stay calm. Explain everything that's happening and remind him why he's there in the first place.

"Dad, we're at the hospital to have a cataract removed from your right eye. You'll be able to see so much better afterward. Isn't that great? Right now the nurse is going to give you some eye drops to help numb your eye, okay? I'll be right here with you."

If Dad is to undergo general anesthesia, you can probably leave him in the hands of the staff once he's sedated. Before you leave, however, you make a point of leaving a songbook on Dad's gurney and announcing clearly,

"If Dad gets agitated, I suggest you start singing "Home on the Range" or "You Are My Sunshine." Those are his favorites."

You're likely to get some startled looks from the staff, but keep a straight face. You'll get their attention and remind them that he has dementia, and they're guaranteed to fetch you as soon as he starts coming out of the anesthesia. It works every time!

(Also: Baby Talk, Communication, Comprehension, Conversations, Empathy, Honesty, Humor, Laughter)

---

*You can turn painful situations around through laughter.
If you can find humor in anything ...you can survive.*
                                                        -Bill Cosby

HUMOR

Mom has always had a good sense of humor, though now she has some difficulties with the language. Her jokes and funny sayings are sometimes a little difficult to understand, but you make a point of reacting to her little asides as you would expect her to react to yours. She occasionally misses the subtlety of some jokes, so try to be more obvious and basic with your amusing remarks. When you share a good laugh it can bring you closer together and give you some relief in situations that can otherwise be trying for both of you. You want to maintain her dignity at all times by making sure that you laugh with her, not at her.

You can use gross exaggerations, silly remarks, self-deprecation, or tell her stories about a faux pas of your own, real or fabricated. It helps her to hear that you make silly mistakes, too.

You can get a quick laugh by giving ridiculous choices (with a straight face, of course).

Goofy choices at the ice cream parlor:

"Which flavor would you like? Chocolate or salami?"

Silly choices in planning the day:
"Ok, we have two choices. You tell me what you want to do: we can spend the rest of the day at home sitting in our chairs staring into space and twiddling our thumbs OR we can go on an amazingly wonderful excursion to that new book store downtown followed by a cup of cappuccino at the coffee bar. I know this is a tough decision. Do you need some more time to think about it?"

Duh!
"Let's hit the road. . . . but the road hasn't done anything, and besides it would hurt us more than it would hurt the road. So maybe we should just drive on it instead."

"You look as happy as a clam! . . . By the way, how can you tell when a clam's happy?

Oops:
"I'm thinking, I'm thinking. Can you hear the wheels turning? Hear that noise! Oh no, I guess that noise is a lawn mower. Oops!"

"Here we are, all belted into the car, ready to go, now if I can only find the keys. Have you noticed it helps to use keys when you drive a car?"

You offer Mom a piece of chocolate and very seriously explain to her how chocolate can improve her health,

"Here's a piece of chocolate for you. Did I tell you that chocolate raises the endorphin level in our bodies? Endorphins are important for our immune systems and help keep us healthy. Now, you have to think of this chocolate as medicine. You're not supposed to enjoy medicine, you know. You're not enjoying it, are you?"

Humor can help both of you over many of the bumps you may experience in your daily lives.

(Also: Affections, Attitude, Empathy, Laughter)

Laughter is the shortest distance between two people.
-Victor Borge

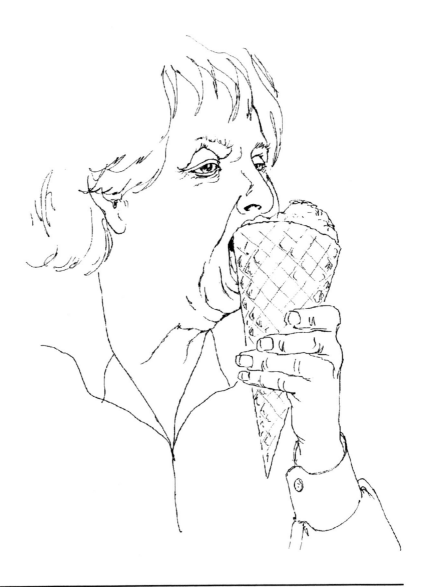

Success is living up to your potential. That's all.
Wake up with a smile and go after life ...
Live it, enjoy it, taste it, smell it, feel it.

-Joe Kapp

i

IDENTIFICATION

It's a good idea to get an identification bracelet for Mom that states her Alzheimer's condition, as well as any allergies she might have. Have it inscribed with her name, your address, and your phone number. It'll help if strangers encounter her wandering about, or if they try to intervene and you need to quickly explain Mom's situation to them.

Medical identifications are available both as bracelets and necklaces. Since a necklace could be caught on something, we consider a bracelet the safer choice for a confused person.

You can find order forms at your local pharmacy or check our list of references. Ask for a "medical alert" bracelet.

The Alzheimer's Association has a program named Safe Return, which combines ID bracelets with a hotline to facilitate uniting you with Mom when she has wandered off.

(Also: Aggression, Conversations, Safe Return, Appendix)

INCONTINENCE

Attitude

Since we were first potty trained, we've been conditioned to view urination and defecation as embarrassing or disgusting, even though they are functions as natural to the body as breathing. We've spent our lives being careful not to soil ourselves. From early infancy it's been drummed into our heads that we have to use the toilet and wipe ourselves well. Mom still has those same needs to be clean, but doesn't always remember until it's too late. It's important for her to continue using the toilet by herself as much as she can, even though she gets upset when she has an accident. Her short-term memory loss may actually be the cause, because she can no longer remember when she last used the bathroom. She doesn't think of it until her body has the urge and then it may be too late.

Mom may understand and accept that she needs a panty shield, but she may still feel upset and ashamed if she's had an accident. If you decide it's necessary to use incontinence aids, please call them "pads" or "briefs," never "diapers," a word that is demeaning to an adult. It may be inconvenient at times, but you need to change her pad as soon as it's soiled.

You can establish a routine of taking her to the toilet frequently and at specific times: after meals, before leaving the house, before a nap or bedtime, and right after she gets up. You may need to accompany her to the toilet and coach her through the motions to make sure she actually relieves herself. It's also beneficial to learn her body language so you can recognize a sign that she needs to go to the toilet. She might suddenly seem distracted or maybe she starts to twist in her seat; both might be signals that she needs to go to the bathroom.

When you're going to be away from home, it's a good idea to place a shield or pad in her panties if you think you may have difficulties finding access to a toilet.

If Mom's accidents become frequent, you may want to look into the variety of protective products available on the market. A heavy-duty shield or "half brief" may be all Mom needs. Keep in mind that most "full briefs" are taped in place at the waist and are almost impossible for Mom to remove by herself.

Accidents

Mom's just had an "accident" and she's distraught. After lunch, you had taken her to the restroom, but now that you're coming out of the movies, you see that her pants have a wet spot. Mom's very agitated, complaining loudly that someone put the wrong pants on her and she's rubbing at the spot frantically. You calmly lead her to the restroom (which you notice always seems to be at the opposite end of the building).

"Mom, I need to go to the bathroom so why don't you come with me. We brought another pair of underwear so you can change into them and that'll make you feel much better. This spot will dry really fast and as soon as we get home, I'll help you change into another pair of pants."

As you take your time chatting with Mom along the way, you notice that as long as you stay calm, others pay little attention to the two of you. You're also letting Mom know by your tone and attitude that you care more about her than any of those strangers around you. You don't rush her. When you get her to the toilet, you remain cheerfully composed as you clean her up and help her change into clean underwear.

It may an awkward maneuver for you with strangers all around, but maintain your nonchalant attitude as you change her half brief. It's easier to accomplish this while she's still sitting on the toilet. With tiny stalls typical of a public restroom, you'll probably have to keep the door open to accommodate both you and Mom. Hopefully a handicap stall is available, which will give you more privacy. Talk her through the motions in a normal tone of voice. This may be hard the first time, but remember that this is something that can happen to anybody and your only concern is for Mom's wellbeing. Other people in the restroom may surprise you with comments like:

"I hope someone'll be there for me when I need it."

Bedtime
Although Dad uses the toilet by himself during the day, you still have to remind him to go. Even before it becomes a necessity, cover Dad's mattress with a full plastic sheet. Later, when it does become essential, place an "under pad" on top of the sheet. If possible, use a comforter in a duvet cover instead of blankets and loose sheets that can become a tangled net for a confused person in a rush to reach the bathroom. Most importantly, don't give him anything to drink for the last two hours before his bedtime. Have Dad wear a "half brief" that will handle small accidents. Use them in place of his shorts because they pull on and off easily. Though he's now set for bed, you'll probably still have to remind him to use the toilet sometime during the course of the night. If you're too late and he has an accident, kindly reassure him,

"Oh, well. Anyone can have an accident, Dad."

Talk cheerfully about something else while you change the sheets and his pajamas. Try to stay positive, even if it's three o'clock in the morning.

Dad may eventually need to advance to "full briefs." There are a few brands featuring an elastic waist band, though the most common "full briefs" are taped closed, which makes them just about impossible for Dad to pull down and up by himself. If he wears them at night, he'll need your help to remove them.

Products
There's a bewildering variety of products on the market, from menstrual pads to full briefs. They basically fall into these categories:

* Minimum protection: panty liners, panty shields
* Medium protection: half briefs, with elastic fasteners or elastic waistbands.
* Maximum protection: full briefs (S, M, L, XL) taped or an elasticized waist for a better fit.
* Under-pads: Protection for beds, chairs, or car seats.

These products are readily available at your local supermarket, drugstore, or membership stores. Local home-health stores and some mail-order houses sell the more specialized versions.

(Also: Attitude, Bathroom, Communication, Dignity, Humor)

We have one simple rule here:
Be kind.
     -Sam Jaffe, "Lost Horizon"

INDEPENDENCE

Dad had been living in his own house before he came to live with you, when it became clear that he could no longer manage on his own. He's not happy with the arrangement. All his adult life he was self-employed and very much in control of his own life, but now he's living in your house, by your rules and routines, so it's a hard transition for him. You've been conscious of this and make sure that he has as much independence as possible. You continually give him choices and routinely ask for his opinions. You're trying to make him feel as if he's a part of day-to-day decisions. You can give him jurisdiction over his living area even if it's only his bedroom. Let him decide where and how things are arranged. When you have to clean it, try to do so either when he's not there, or ask him to help you, or offer to give him a hand.

"Dad, you said you'd like me to help clean your room. I can help you this afternoon, I hope that's all right with you."

If he's agreeable, you can act as his assistant.

"I brought the vacuum cleaner. Would you like me to run it, or do you want to do it yourself?"

(Also: Dignity, Empathy, Privacy, Personal Space)

Take the gentle path.
-George Herbert

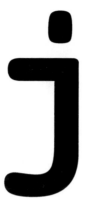

JOURNALS

It's a good idea to keep diaries or journals, some for practical reasons, others for fun and family history. Keep track of Dad's physical and mental conditions if he's on a special diet or medication. Some medications have potentially serious side effects and the more information about his reactions that you can bring to his doctors, the better they'll be able to adjust the dose or find safer alternatives, if necessary.

You also may want to keep some kind of diary of your daily activities, even if it's only a line or two in a daybook. This helps you keep track of his favorite meals and places to go, fun games, and entertaining stories. If you enjoy writing, you can keep a journal of Dad's stories or of humorous experiences you've shared. This will give you a priceless record of the time you spend together.

When Dad has moments of clarity, take advantage of them and encourage him to talk about his memories. You can encourage him to write an "autobiography" with your assistance. Augment it with your own notes. You may have heard these stories many times before, but they take on a special meaning when you write them down. These projects should be fun, not chores.

(Also: Medication, Recording Memories)

It doesn't matter who my father was; it matters who I remember he was.

           -Anne Sexton

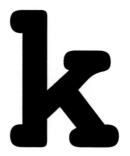

KITCHEN

Dad never came near the kitchen during your growing-up years. As a matter of fact, he barely knew where it was, so when you suggest that he help you with the cooking, he's incredulous. But since he's been having trouble eating lately, you figure that this may be one way to get him interested in food again. You start by having him sit on a stool in the kitchen to watch you as you cook. You engage in a running commentary of the cooking process. Have him get involved, one small step at a time.

"Dad, would you mind cutting up this banana for me? Small slices will be just fine, about a quarter of an inch."

Play it by ear and be sure he's using tools that are safe for him. Let him set his own pace as much as possible and let his involvement develop slowly. It's important that he enjoys himself and who knows, his eating habits might even improve.

Mom was known as quite a gourmet cook in her former social circle. You'd been so intimidated by her skills that you stayed as far away from the kitchen as possible and missed out on learning some of her finest culinary tricks. Since you've grown up, however, you've managed to become a fairly decent cook, even a subscriber to Gourmet Magazine.

Mom had several near disasters with fire and knives in her own kitchen while she was still living by herself, which is one the reasons why she's now living with you. Of course it's been frustrating for her, because she has no memory of her accidents, so she thinks that you're just being mean or jealous by keeping her out of the kitchen.

Mom has been sitting with you in the kitchen while you cook, but she drives you crazy with her constant comments. Nothing you do is "her way," which of course in her mind is the only right way. Before you explode in exasperation, consider getting her safely involved in the cooking process. Start by putting her in charge of the salads, cutting up soft fruit and vegetables, or mixing batters. Most importantly, ask for her opinion and advice and listen patiently to her explanation, however jumbled and nonsensical it might be. In the end you'll do it your own way, but it makes her feel good to think you've followed her directions.

As you open a can of mushroom soup, you can say:

"Mom, you used to make an incredible sauce for the roast chicken. I'd like to make it tonight. Let me see . . . I start by heating up the stock. Does this look right?"

"They should be the right way. One, two, three, four. People think they can have two. That's right."

You have no idea what she's talking about, but continue as if she makes perfect sense as you pretend to sprinkle seasonings into the pot:

". . . and then I add these fresh herbs. Let me see... we have thyme and rosemary and your secret ingredient. . . . What was it again?"

"Eight, nine, ten, eleven, twelve. . ."

"I think it's a dash of nutmeg, right? Twelve? I don't know. That sounds like too much. What do you think? Maybe it is two dashes. One – two. Oh yes, now that smells just like your famous sauce. You've always been an excellent cook and I have so much to learn from you. Thank you so much for helping me out, Mom."

Since Mom likes to count these days, you're getting her attention by counting with her, and you make her feel good by giving her a compliment.

If Mom likes to fiddle around in the kitchen, you can set aside a drawer for her for tools and other things that she likes to work with. (Use childproof safety locks on cabinets with tools that are not safe.)

You can also support her interest in cooking by helping her create her own recipe collection. Even if she's no longer able to cook on her own, she'll probably enjoy rifling through cooking magazines. You can encourage her to cut out recipes and paste them into a scrapbook. This can provide her with a diversion when you need it.

(Also: Fixations, Home Safety, Honesty, Loving Lies, Projects, Personal Space)

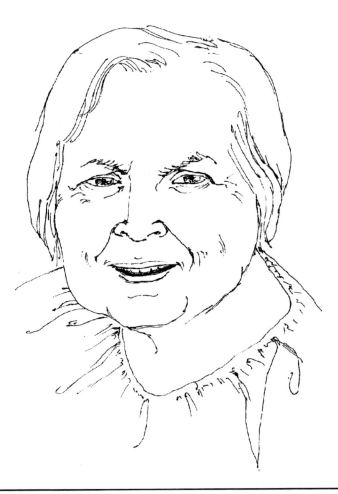

The discovery of a new dish does more for the happiness of the human race than the discovery of a star.
                    -Jean Anthelme Brillat-Savarin

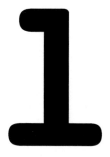

LAUGHTER

Laughter, hugs, and chocolate raise the levels of endorphins in our bodies and boost our immune systems, so they're very powerful healing tools for both you and Mom. Now that her life's getting more confusing, Mom will have a much easier time if you can help her approach daily life with a light heart and a sense of humor.

Mom will probably provide you with plenty of good chuckles, but you don't want to make her self-conscious. Be sure to laugh with her, never at her, and try to find something in yourself that you can both laugh at as well.

Laughter will help ease your own stress and it also can help Mom realize that you don't take her mistakes seriously, so why should she?

Since Mom's forgetting a lot these days, she may enjoy the irony of you forgetting something too.

"You're not going to believe this, Mom. This morning, I could not remember where I had put my glasses. I looked all over the house for them. I looked everywhere. Do you know where I found them? Right on top of my head! They had been there all along, but I didn't realize it until I passed the mirror and saw my own reflection out of the corner of my eye. Boy, did I laugh at myself!"

Remind her that you and she suffer "senior moments" while everyone else just plain forgets.

The best laughs come from your own experiences. Look back at your own life for funny stories. You can keep a log of the stories that bring Mom the most joy and repeat them often,

"Did I ever tell you about the . . ."

You can also start a collection of humorous books and videos, though that may be easier said than done. Unfortunately much contemporary adult humor tends to be mean-spirited. You might find some humor books at the library, especially in the children's department. Also, look for classic movies and comedy videos.

(Also: Attitude, Empathy, Exercise, Games, Humor, Word Games)

Time spent laughing is time spent with the Gods.
-Japanese Proverb

LAURELS

Mom once spent a lot of time as a community volunteer. She baked cookies for the PTA, knitted booties for unwed mothers, and she led a Girl Scout troop, rarely getting the recognition she so rightly deserved. She shrugged it off at the time, but now it's all coming back to her. It took you a while to figure out what she was talking about because she'd get very agitated and say, almost in tears,

"All the work I did for them and they never even said thank you. I'm never gonna do anything for them again!"

When you finally realize what she's talking about and you try to explain to her that it took place thirty or forty years ago, she instead directs her anger at you. You realize that you can praise her all you want, but it will not have the same effect as recognition from others. You can present her with an award retroactively. You can use our standard "Award," purchase one at a stationery store, or create your own, but make sure that it looks professional and send it to her through the mail. If there were several deeds she should have received recognition for, every few weeks send a different award for each one.

In your everyday conversations you can remind her of the positive things she's done in her life. Recount her good deeds and accomplishments, and pass on any praise you remember hearing from other people. This can boost Mom's sense of wellbeing and self-worth, especially if she is nonverbal. Try to avoid too much embellishment, however, because she may have recalled a lot more than you realize.

Dad loved baseball when he was a kid and you'd heard about his pitching skills for as long as you can remember. When he talks about it now, it's with longing and sadness that he'll never win that trophy that he worked so hard for, all those years ago. You can have a trophy or plaque made for him. Make sure it looks authentic.

(Also: Dignity, Memories)

AWARD
OF
EXCELLENCE

Let it be known that

_____

has always been a valued member of our community and has contributed countless hours without any expectation of rewards.

We hereby acknowledge our indebtedness.

_____

LISTENING

Dad's delighted when you really "listen" to him. His words don't make much sense to you, but by watching his body language and listening for verbal clues, you're able to get a sense of his intent.

"It is so grompsy, when they tool it."

You respond with,

"It sounds as if you've given this some thought."

He glows with pleasure, as he says,

"That shilley is loyal, many now."

What's he talking about? You have no idea, so you give him a neutral response:

"That's very interesting."

Then you recall a TV program that he was watching with particular interest the night before.

"Weren't they talking about that on TV last night?"

By making these kinds of comments, you can find yourself engaged in a lengthy "discussion" with a totally delighted Dad. Giving him neutral responses might help you eventually figure out what he's talking about.

Mom's still able to express herself in a somewhat linear fashion, but she's lost a lot of vocabulary so she uses replacement words. You use "active listening" to help her without sounding like you're correcting her.

"The sessie's so much pretty. There was a well one."

"Yes, I agree with you, Mom. That was one of the nicest department stores we've been to in a long time. There was so much to look at. It sounds as if you particularly liked that beige sweater. Do you think we should go back and buy it?"

And if she gets frustrated and dangles half-finished sentences, you gently help her finish them as though it's a perfectly normal thing to do.

"I want to go in ... with the wheels."

You say with a smile,

"The car? Funny you should say that, because I was just about to ask you if you wanted to go for a ride in the car later this afternoon. Great minds think alike, eh?"

(Also: Communication, Comprehension, Discussions, Normal, Questions, Repetitions, Word Substitutions)

Show me a person who has never made a mistake and I'll show you someone who has never achieved much.
-Joan Collins

LOVING LIES

Mom's busy packing her underwear into a shoebox. When you ask her what she's doing, she says,

"Mother's waiting for me. I must go!"

You realize that Mom's thinking of herself as a little kid with a mother waiting at home. If you tried to convince her that she's hallucinating, she might get unnecessarily upset. This is one time when it's okay to use a loving lie. You need to sound believable and sincere and it's important to follow up with some sort of diversion.

"Oh, I'm sorry. I forgot to tell you. Your mother called and said she has a meeting at the church tonight and she wants you to stay here and eat dinner with me."

And then:

"You said earlier you wanted to help me fix dinner. If the offer still stands, I think now is a perfect time. Come, let's go to the kitchen."

Another time, Mom's very agitated,

"Someone stole my favorite beige coat! You just can't trust anybody these days!"

The beige coat had succumbed to the moths by the time you were fourteen, but you calmly respond with:

"We took it to the cleaners this morning. We can pick it up tomorrow, they said. How about wearing your dusty blue jacket today. You look so pretty in that color. "

Then you divert her attention with:

"I wonder if the new Gardening magazine arrived yet. If you have time right now, would you mind checking the mail on the table?"

❧

The loving lie has to be authentic sounding and in character. For example, Dad's friend obsesses about his wife's whereabouts, although she died eight years ago. Someone tells him, "Oh, she went out shopping this afternoon." Rather than being reassured as expected, he reacts with increased agitation. As it turns out, his wife had been a workaholic with so little free time that shopping had become such a rare event that it was reserved just for the two of them to share. When he's told that his wife had gone shopping without him, of course he became upset. That's why a loving lie must accurately relate to the people involved.

@

Mom was a long-standing member of a prominent civic organization. In spite of her shyness, she would often make public appearances on its behalf. This happened so long ago that you have no memory of what she's talking about, when she asks you,

"Where are my notes? What did I do with them? Have you seen them?"

You find a sheet of paper on her nightstand and present it to her, but this only seems to aggravate her more. You search her room while you're searching your brain for a clue as to what she's talking about when she says,

"I can't go before them without my notes."

Ah! A speech! Remembering her occasional experiences as a public speaker, you sit down with her and seriously explain,

"We got a telephone call right before you took your nap. They called and said the event has been postponed until next week. The other two speakers have come down with that flu that's going around. So now you have a whole extra week to worry about it (ha, ha). If you want to rehearse, I'll be glad to be your guinea pig audience."

This is a perfect opportunity to encourage her to talk about her past experiences with civic affairs. Turn on your tape recorder, sit back, and listen. You might learn something new about your Mom at the same time that you're calming her down.

(Also: Communication, Diversions, Empathy, Laurels, Normal, Reality)

The biggest mistake is believing that there is one right way to listen, to talk, to have a conversation – or a relationship.

-Deborah Tannen

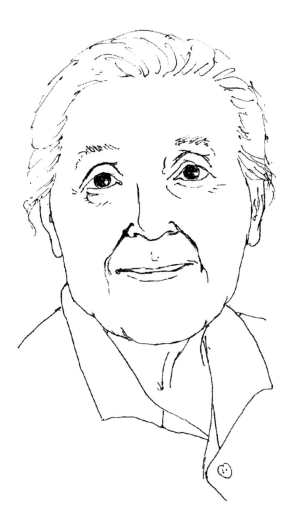

The healthy and strong individual is the one
who asks for help when he needs it.
                                        -Rona Barrett

m

MASSAGE

You share several hugs with Dad throughout the day and give him a casual back scratch now and then. Your touch can be soothing to him when he's agitated. Simply resting your hand on his arm or back can often calm him.

You keep a bottle of lotion handy to massage his hands and occasionally his feet. Not only does this help relieve the dryness in his skin, but it is the easiest way to soothe him and enhance his sense of connection to you. A more elaborate massage can do wonders to make Dad feel good, both physically and mentally. If he's shy because he's never had a massage before, you can use a gradual approach to help him feel more comfortable. Start by massaging his arms and legs until he's more relaxed.

"It feels so good, doesn't it? And for once, something that feels good is good for you! Would you like to try a back massage?"

Ask him to sit on a straight-back chair, facing backward, with his legs straddling the seat and his arms resting on the back of the chair. He can keep his shirt on for the first several rounds. Describe the massage step by step as you stroke his back.

"I'm going to give you a good back massage, Dad. Can you feel how I'm rubbing your back? It's good for your muscles and your circulation. You'll feel so good after this. I guarantee it."

When you sense that he's feeling at ease, you can help him to remove his shirt as you explain what you are going to do. Reiterate how good it will feel. If he's shy, you can emphasize the "medical" necessity and physical benefits as you give him a back massage.

Apply massage oil and lightly stroke his back in large circular moves – very carefully, because elderly bones are fragile and elderly skin bruises easily. A deeper massage for Dad is best left to a professional. If he feels muscle pain or joint aches, it may be time to take him to a massage therapist with a background in geriatrics. Discuss this with his doctor before making a decision.

(Also: Affections, Empathy, Humor, Pain)

There is nothing stronger in the world than gentleness.
-Han Suyin

MEDICATION

Dad has to be on "life-sustaining" medication, so you want him to have the best results with the mildest side effects. It's a good idea to establish a rapport with your pharmacist and request circulars so you can discuss with her any prescriptions and possible alternatives. There's an average of 10,000 prescription drugs on the market at any one time and each comes with a "circular" which is a description of the medication, benefits, side effects, test results, etc., all in the tiniest print. The circulars will be easier for you to read if you make copies of them enlarged to 200%.

There are several excellent publications, written for the public, which review the most popularly prescribed medications. Check your local bookstore.

Mom's doctor has suggested medications to improve her quality of life. Before you commit her to any of these medications, however, you'll want to investigate them thoroughly. Some of them may have very serious, possibly irreversible, side effects. You may also want to look into natural herbal remedies. When you decide a medication is acceptable, keep a journal of Mom's mental and physical condition while she's on it. If you notice a negative reaction in her, you may decide that you're better off handling her conditions without the use of drugs, instead following the methods outlined in this book.

Tip: Keep all medication and chemical substances (including cleaning liquids) securely locked up. Don't keep anything in the bathroom medicine cabinet or under the sink that Mom might mistakenly ingest (sweet smelling liquid soaps, for example.)

(Also: Alternative Remedies, Alzheimer's Disease, Dementia, Pain, Pills)

MEMORIES

Coaching

"Dad, when we visited your sister yesterday, the two of you talked a lot about growing up. I really enjoy it when you talk about your childhood."

Reiterate as much as you can in order to encourage Dad's participation. This might lead him to join in with you because he won't feel pressure to remember anything specific, so his memory may flow more easily. At this point, and with great enthusiasm, he will once again regale you with the same old favorite story. Telling this anecdote gives him such joy, but you fear that you may not be able suppress a howl of "God spare us! Not again." Instead of feigning interest yet one more time, wait for a lull in his story and then redirect him by asking a question that might stimulate a new aspect of the same old saga:

"I wish I'd known your friend. I really enjoy hearing about your experiences with him. I was wondering what other games you played. I'd love to hear about some of your other explorations."

This may trigger additional stories, though it's likely this is the only one about his friend that's left in his memory bank. You might instead ask a general question about a particular period of his life. Talk about your own life, choosing general experiences that might be similar to his. You may learn something new about your Dad, so keep your tape recorder handy, just in case.

"You know, Dad, when I was a teenager, we'd go to King's drive-in just about every Friday after school for hamburgers. I was wondering if you and your friends had a ritual like that?"

You can talk about something that both of you have in common:

"When I was doing the wash this morning I was remembering what it was like to do the laundry before we had a clothes drier. In the winter the sheets would freeze as stiff as boards as soon as we got them on the line. Boy, our hands got cold!"

Or:

"Do you know what I really miss? Listening to the radio! Now everybody watches TV. I loved listening to the radio with you and Mom when I was little. There was a show we all loved to listen to. What was the name of it? Darn it, I don't remember, do you?"

It's reassuring for Dad to hear that you occasionally have problems remembering things. No matter what he recalls, just go along with him, though there's a better chance he'll remember the name of a radio show than his mother's birthplace. You may have been thinking of "The Shadow," but he says "The Jack Benny Show." It doesn't really matter. The important thing is that you can reminisce about good times you've shared.

Pitfalls

You want to stay away from challenging Dad's memory with questions that require specific knowledge.

"What's the name of the town where your mother was born and grew up?"

"How many children do you have?"

"Where did you live?"

"How old were you?"

You may find it disturbing that Dad can't even remember his own children but you'll find that if you force the issue, you'll only make him depressed and unhappy.

"Don't you remember . . .?" and "Do you remember . . .?" questions may trigger a panic in Dad when he realizes that he can't remember and he thinks he ought to. In other words, these kinds of questions emphasize his dementia.

Instead, you can start his reminiscing by recounting the event or person. Go into details until you sense recognition on his part.

"It was some time ago, so you may not remember . . ."

"You met this person months ago and there were a lot of other people around at the time, so I'd be surprised if you'd remember."

You give Dad an opening and take the pressure off him.

Exceptions:

"Do you remember high school? Halloween? Ford Model-T's?"

These are such broad subjects that he's apt to remember something and if he doesn't offer a response, it doesn't matter, because even he's aware that this is inconsequential chitchat.

(Also: Communication, Listening, No!, Normal, Questions, Recording Memories)

I have spread my dreams under your feet;
Tread softly because you tread on my dreams.
-William Butler Yeats

MONEY

You've handled Dad's money for some time now, but give him a few bills and some change to keep in his wallet so he can pay for small purchases now and again. Money has been an important symbol of his self-respect throughout his productive life.

The two of you are standing at the checkout stand when he looks at the few bills in his wallet and becomes very agitated:

"Who took my money? Someone took my money! I had all my money in here. Now it's gone. Who took all my money?"

You take his arm gently and say,

"May I see your wallet, Dad? I see . . . looks like you have about $15.00. I think that's all you decided to bring today. Yesterday you put the rest of your money in the bank for safe-keeping."

"I don't remember doing that."

"Yesterday was such a busy day, I'd also forgotten about the bank until you brought it up just now. I'll go ahead and pay our bill and you can pay me back later when we go back to the bank, okay?"

If Dad keeps obsessing about his money, you can arrange to have him receive a "paycheck" in the mail every Friday. It's a wonderful ego booster for him. You can then offer to "deposit" his "check" at the bank and later tear it up. In the meantime you can have a "bank book" to show him the balance of his earnings.

Mom loves carrying her purse. She often fills it with an odd assortment of things: a tube of toothpaste, some old greeting cards, and a solitary sock. Sometimes you slip a few bills into the wallet before taking her out.

You've just finished lunch at a local café. Mom insists on treating you, but you've forgotten to give her some money today. It's tempting to remind her just how well you have been handling her bank account all these years, but you resist.

"Oh, Mom, I couldn't let you do that. You treated the last time we went to lunch, so now it's my turn."

You can take advantage of the situation and give her a compliment that will help to divert her attention:

"You're such a generous person. I'm so lucky to be your daughter. You have taught me so much with your many examples of kindness."

(Also: Diversions, Independence, Loving Lies)

Change is inevitable - except from a vending machine.
- Robert C. Gallagher

MOVIES

Going to the movies has always been a favorite pastime of yours and you've missed it since Mom's been living with you. One afternoon you can't find someone to stay with Mom so you decide to take her to the movies with you, though you're worried that she won't be able to follow the story line and might not enjoy it. She's felt anxious in crowded places lately, so you feel concerned, even as you buy the matinee tickets.

Mom, however, is quite excited as she walks into the theater lobby. After a trip to the restroom, you make your way to your seats in the nearly empty theater. The previews confuse her, so you have to remind her that the movie hasn't started yet.

When it finally begins you discreetly observe her as she watches it and you're pleasantly surprised at her attention. She's enjoying this! Afterwards, when you try to talk about the plot, she has no idea what you're talking about and yet, when you ask her if she liked going to the movie and would like to come back, she responds in enthusiastic agreement.

There's something special about watching a film in a theater with a large screen and big sound. Mom may not be able to follow the story line, but don't be surprised if she reacts to the overall "quality" of the picture. If the characters are well written and the actors convincing, she will likely enjoy the experience, even if she doesn't remember the plot. Some of us forget the plots of many of the movies we've enjoyed; Mom just forgets a lot sooner – like the moment she leaves the theater.

Mom may have a hard time following a movie on a small television screen with all the distractions present in a home setting, but a movie theater is an exciting and magical place that commands her full attention.

Recommendations

You're better off taking Mom to family films, human-interest dramas, and love stories, especially if she hasn't been to the movies in a while. Films made for general audiences are usually easier to watch because the dialog tends to be clear and the story lines are simple. Some cartoons may be violent and mean, although they have the advantage of being obviously fictitious. Mom may be offended that you've taken her to a kiddy show.

Current action films are so realistically violent that they'd easily upset Mom's confused mind.

Unfortunately contemporary comedies are often very physical and mean-spirited, with a lot of sarcasm or cruelty. We might all laugh at a man slipping on a banana peel in a movie, only because we know that he doesn't really get hurt. Dad, however, may not "know" this anymore because of his dementia, so it's not only not funny, it may even be disturbing to him. Recent popular comedies featuring the trials and tribulations of old folks may be hilarious to a younger crowd, but much of this humor is based on the presumption that the frailties of old age are intrinsically amusing. When you are old, however, you certainly don't see it that way.

Select movies that you yourself want to see. Your enjoyment will rub off on her.

(Also: Comprehension, Reality)

MUSIC

The use of music can be a great aid in your daily routines. There is a wide variety of music available that is designed to aid in mood relaxation and elevation. If Dad is agitated, try playing one of these tapes or CDs in the background while you try to figure out what's bothering him. You can use mellow music to help him relax before bedtime and you can use nostalgic big band music to elevate his mood when he's down.

You've invited a few friends to a small dinner party, the first sort of formal event you've hosted since Mom has been living with you. She has been doing her best to be of help in the kitchen all afternoon, but you're so used to cooking alone that you spend most of your time trying to find something for her to do. After a couple of hours of this, your dinner is running late, you're feeling testy, and Mom is quite agitated. In your calmest voice you try to tell her that you have everything under control, but she reacts with obvious rejection; she feels useless and is near tears. Running out of projects in the kitchen, you walk her into the dining room as you attempt to convince her that she's the only one who could possibly set the table to perfection. She's grumbling, and mumbling in protest.

"You just don't like my cooking, do you? I remember when you were a little kid, you'd spit out your food. I just can't do anything right, can I? I hate it here. I'm going home tomorrow!"

You're doing your best to stay calm through this tirade. You have to admit that it hurts. You know that arguing with her is hopeless, so you instead turn to the stereo, play one of the

Chopin CDs you had chosen for the evening and return to the kitchen, leaving Mom to her angry protesting. After a few minutes you realize she's quiet, so you sneak a peak and see her sitting in the big easy chair in front of the stereo, her eyes closed and a faint smile on her face. She's positively beatific sitting there. You've remembered just how powerful music can be as you silently thank Chopin and his colleagues and return to chopping the garlic.

Dad has been having bouts of depression and loneliness. At times he's hallucinating that your mother's waiting for him and when you tell him she's been dead for fifteen years, he either gets angry or he's withdrawn and won't eat. You've discovered that the "cure" to this miserable state is playing his collection of oldies like Jimmie Dorsey and Duke Ellington as background while you sit with him for a few minutes and listen to him talk about the early days with your mother. You then follow up with the gentle sounds of Brahms, so by the time bedtime comes around, you're both feeling mellow and ready for a restful and contented sleep.

Music can bring joy, peace, positive energy, or it can put you into a state of aggravation or nervousness. Music is so powerful in the lives of human beings that the sense of music is apparently the last of our senses to go. You want to keep that in mind when you come to the point of helping Mom through the last days of her life. You can play her favorite music to help her feel at peace.

(Also: Death and Dying, Exercise, Singing)

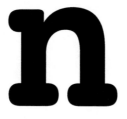

NEIGHBORHOOD FLYER

Mom has started wandering. The other day the two you got separated at the mall. You were beside yourself until a security guard located her. Since that occurrence, you have posted signs on your exits: "DO NOT GO OUT THIS DOOR" and you've ordered an identification bracelet for her. Even with these precautions, there's still a possibility that Mom will wander off. Mom looks perfectly normal, so it's not obvious to strangers that she needs help.

If you live on a typical street or in an apartment building, you may be acquainted with your immediate neighbors, but probably few people beyond that. Still, the neighborhood pulled often together to help look for a lost dog or cat.

It may be worth distributing a flyer to alert the neighborhood of her condition. You can make up your own or use our example:

(Also: Identification, Safe Return, Wandering)

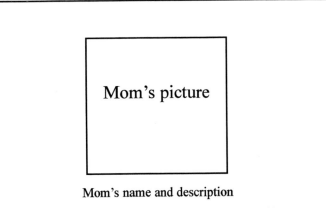

Mom's name and description

Dear Neighbor,

My mother and I live in your neighborhood. Mother has Alzheimer's disease and is often very confused. If you see her alone on the street, please help us in one of the following ways:

Mom wears a Medical Alert bracelet with our phone number.

If we don't answer the phone, we're out looking for her. Please leave your phone number and address on our voice mail and we will be right over to get her.

If you're not comfortable with any of the above, please call the police right away with the location where you last saw her and the direction in which she was headed.

We realize this may be an imposition and we appreciate in advance any assistance you give us.

Thank you.

Your name

P.S. Mom likes strawberry jam, tea with a half-teaspoon of sugar, ice cream, and potato chips. She loves children and cats.

No!

The one word that can create the most resistance between you and your Mom is "No!" Even in the mildest crisis, you'll find that using the word to stop a behavior only succeeds in causing more confusion for your Mom. The meaning of the word often doesn't register with her at that moment, only the strident tone of your voice. It doesn't stop her from doing what she's doing, it merely agitates or startles her. Instead of reacting by saying "No!," try gently, but quickly, interrupting what she's doing in order to defuse the situation.

Mom is standing at the kitchen counter putting the finishing touches on the dinner salad. She reaches into the refrigerator and pulls out a carton of chocolate soy milk and starts to pour it, thinking it's salad dressing. Your instinct is to yell "No!" but you resist and go quickly to her. If you reach her in time, you can discreetly stop her pouring by putting your hand under the carton as you say,

"Oops, Mom, I think you found the wrong bottle. You told me you wanted to use ranch dressing tonight. It's in that white bottle in the back of the fridge. Do you see it?"

If you don't get there in time, you can use a diversion with her while you try to salvage your salad.

"Do you have any more energy left, Mom? You've been working so hard, but I sure could use your help setting the table. I'll be glad to take care of the vegetables."

Try to avoid a "No!" reaction, even when the situation is more serious. Mom has placed a potholder on top of a burner in the mistaken belief that it's a teakettle. She's about to turn on the fire. You envision your house going up in flames, so your instincts are to scream "No!" at her. Instead, you take a breath as you dash to her side and quickly retrieve the potholder. Put your arms around her and take another deep breath as you say as calmly as you can,

"What a good idea, I could use a cup of tea right now. Do you want to fill the kettle? What flavor should we have?"

This incident, by the way, is a warning to pay attention to kitchen safety. You might want to take the knobs off the stove so this doesn't happen again.

You're learning to be mindful of how you phrase questions to Mom. If you ask a question that puts Mom's memory on the spot, such as "Do you remember how many kids Aunt Emma had?" you'll probably get a response of "No" simply because she's not sure what you're talking about.

"Yes" and "no" type questions are great when you want Mom to participate in a casual chat, but if you need her to do something, ask your question in a way that predicts the answer. If you ask, "Do you want to take a bath?" you're most likely to get a firm "No!" Try using a more subtle approach:

"Mom, I have something to show you. – Here, let me help you out of the chair. – There! – Now we're going down this way. You and I went to the store yesterday and you bought a fluffy green towel and you made me promise you that you could use it today after your bath. See, now doesn't that towel feel soft?"

(Also: Bath Time, Coaching, Communication, Diversions, Home Safety, Normal, Questions)

NORMAL

"But she seems so normal."

You've gotten used to hearing this when people learn that Mom has been diagnosed with Alzheimer's disease.

If you were to ask her, she may acknowledge a bit of a memory problem, but other than that she considers herself perfectly normal.

This feeling of "normal" is at the core of our self-awareness. We are all different, of course, and can only view the world from our individual perspectives that are shaped by genetics, environment, and culture. Most of us do our best to be empathetic, but everything we think and do is always measured against our core self-image.

Wouldn't you still consider yourself "normal" if you had a broken arm, missing teeth, arthritis, or diabetes? Now, how about baldness, hearing impairment, or sight impairment? So why should you feel any different with Alzheimer's? We all think of ourselves as normal, including the memory impaired. Mom has Alzheimer's disease, but she's not "sick" as such. Rather, she's in an altered state of mind and is not cognizant of the dramatic changes in her personality. However, the world feels more and more confusing to her.

Mom's behavior may seem odd to you at times, but keep in mind that she still thinks of herself as normal. From her point of view it's the circumstances that are strange and she's merely reacting to them. You can help her maintain her self-confidence by addressing her with a normal attitude and tone of voice.

Mom gets lost going to the bathroom after having had no problems for months. She has lapsed into a different reality and she's back in her childhood home where the bathroom was on the opposite end of the house. In her mind she's normal, but the bathroom location has changed. You can help her by relating to the "normal" in her and acknowledge her reality. Let her know that forgetting can happen to anybody:

"Where is it? I can't find it, they moved it. Where's the bathroom?"

"Come with me, I'll be glad to show you. – I think I know how you feel. Sometimes I wake up in the morning and everything looks weird to me because I was dreaming about my old house right before I woke up. It's such a strange feeling, isn't it? But rest assured, the bathroom is right down this hallway."

You can strengthen this feeling by asking for her suggestions on things that don't tax her memory. You can make up a "problem" and ask her advice on gardening, cooking, or relationships. She might just surprise you. She may have lost a lot of her memory, but her core personality hasn't changed and her common sense is still there to some degree. It's important to her self-confidence that you value her opinion. – You don't have to follow her advice any more now than you did when you were a teenager.

(Also Empathy, Loving Lies, Questions, Transitions)

The only normal people are the ones we don't know very well.
–Anonymous

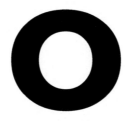

OBSESSIVE BEHAVIOR

Mom has developed a fascination with counting. She will count the steps as you walk with her and she'll count when you help her get dressed. She starts counting whenever she's not engaged in conversation. Rather than letting yourself get exasperated by this repetitive numbers game, try to cheerfully join in:

"Do you think we'll reach a hundred before we get to the door? I bet we will. You're already at eighty-four, aren't you? Eighty-five, eighty-six, . . ."

You're eating lunch when she says,

"Sixty-two, sixty-three, seventy-five percent."

You can join in with:

"Seventy-five percent? You know, I had only gotten it up to sixty percent. Boy, you're way ahead of me. But I trust your judgment. You've always been so good at numbers. When I was a kid, you'd help me with my math. I wonder if I would have learned any of it if it hadn't been for you."

Who knows why she has this obsession with numbers, but try to take it in stride. There's nothing wrong in Mom doing it, and in fact, it seems to bring her some kind of peace.

(Also: Diversions, Fixations, Word Substitutions)

If you think you can, you can.
And if you think you can't, you're right.
-Mary Kay Ash

OUTINGS

The last time you saw this much of your community was on the elementary school field trips you took when you were nine or ten. Lately you and Dad have been exploring museums, galleries, libraries, and parks. You aim for one outing a week, often going back to favorite haunts.

Drives

You had planned to take Mom to the library today, but now you realize that there just isn't enough time. She's getting restless so you decide to take her for a short drive instead.

"Mom, I'm getting cabin fever. I need to get out of here. How about you? Wanna go for a drive with me?"

Your trip doesn't have to be a long one to be enjoyable. You can take a leisurely drive around the neighborhood and talk about what you see along the way: grass that's too high and needs cutting, big blue flowers or small yellow ones, a cute little dog, or a garbage truck making its rounds. You're cruising along in a relaxed and carefree atmosphere. Mom's chatting happily and though she may not make much sense, you enthusiastically go along with her conversation.

Once in a while let Mom decide where to go. As you get ready to pull out into the street, ask her as you point to the directions:

"Okay Mom, which way do we go, right or left?"

As you approach the first major intersection ask her again:

"Now, when we get to the light, do we go this way or that? Or straight ahead?"

You may end up driving in circles, but so what? At least it's not boring and Mom becomes empowered by making the decisions. Keep it up as long as she enjoys it, though it's likely that she'll tire soon. When you get home and talk about your outing, you can honestly give her the credit for an enjoyable trip:

"Wow, what a trip! It was so much fun having you lead the way. I had a great time. I got to see streets I didn't even know existed. We got to see those beautiful flowers. They reminded me of our garden when I was little. Except I think your flowers were much prettier. You have always been an excellent gardener."

Mom loves to listen to you talk about your childhood when you include stories about her. Mom may not be able to remember specific events, so you avoid asking her directly: "Do you remember. . . ?" Instead, try a story telling approach:

"Speaking of flowers, you know what one of my very early memories is? The time when I decided to "help" you with the tulips, so I went out and picked off the heads of a whole bunch of them and brought them to you. – How old was I? Three or four maybe? – And you were so sweet and thanked me and said something about letting the other tulips stay in the ground for a while longer. What blows me away, Mom, is that you didn't even get mad. I mean, I had just ruined your finest flowerbed! Every time I see a tulip, that memory comes back to me. You probably don't even remember, do you? But you know how I'm always trying to save half-wilted plants from certain demise. Do you suspect I'm trying to make up for what I did to your tulips?"

Galleries

Mom loves art, so you explore local art museums and galleries on your outings with her. When you find a gallery that Mom is particularly fond of, you can initiate a conversation with the staff and talk to them about Mom's dementia. The next time you visit, their recognition of her can make her feel important and knowledgeable.

If you visit a gallery in the mornings you can usually have the place to yourselves, which gives the two of you plenty of time for arts discussions. Ask the gallery director for past show announcements that you can later use for collage projects or in Mom's scrapbooks. If Mom has a workspace at home and her interest is art, the announcements can help fill her file.

Libraries

Mom still thinks of herself as an avid reader, though she usually doesn't get past the first page, which she reads over and over again. A trip to the library can become a favorite outing and help fill her day. If she has trouble accessing the shelves, you can find her a comfortable chair in one of the reading rooms and go find books for her. If she loves gardens, find her a beautiful picture book of flowers, but be sure to open it to a picture page, or she might not get past the opening text. This would be a good time to reminisce with her. She probably remembers working in her own garden. If she doesn't, you can still entertain yourselves by creating richly detailed stories of fantasy gardens.

While at the library, check out music books for your sing-alongs, how-to books on crafts projects, and books of poetry and short stories to read out loud. In addition, many libraries have excellent video collections available for checkout from National Geographic and Public Television. Most libraries also have books on tape, which Mom may enjoy if she can still follow a good story line.

Museums

You and Dad have discovered a local museum that offers free admission to seniors one day a week. Fortunately, wheelchairs are available so that when Dad is tired you can wheel him around. Reassure him that this has nothing to do with his being disabled:

"Aren't we lucky? Here's a wheelchair we can use. Oh, I know you don't really need it, but this is such a big place and there's so much to see. This way you don't have to use up all your energy walking around."

You wheel him to the exhibits you know that he'd be particularly interested in. You may end up looking at only one exhibit the entire afternoon because you're giving him all the time he needs to discuss whatever you are admiring. We often feel the pressure to look at every single thing in a museum, so at first you may get restless with this limited approach. You're not there for information or education; you're there for sheer pleasure, so do what feels right for Dad.

Picnics

You and Dad often talk about the wonderful annual family picnics of his childhood. Of course in the reminiscing only the pleasures are remembered, like Grandma's potato salad and Aunt Ella's peach pie. Miraculously forgotten are the ants, flies, frequent cloudbursts, and running for cover. In Dad's mind a picnic is still the ultimate outing, so the two of you spend a lot of good times making picnic plans and on your drives you often look for perfect locations. One beautiful summer day, you fill your picnic basket with a checkered table cloth and a couple of brightly colored plastic plates, but you pack only a bottle of juice and a few crackers, because you want to make the picnic short and sweet. Aside from the usual discomforts of flies and wind, picnic benches are uncomfortable and very hard on elderly bottoms. All too often the thought of a picnic is far better than the real thing, but a short ten-minute picnic can bring you hours of fond memories later. You can drive past your picnic location on later drives and relive it:

"Look, Dad, there's our favorite picnic bench in the shade of that big tree. We had such a good time there and we should have another picnic soon, don't you think?"

The next picnic may not take place until next summer, but you can still talk about it and plan it in the meantime. Use the idea of picnics in your fantasy games on cold winter days when you are housebound. Get as elaborate as you can in your descriptions as you "plan" and encourage him to come up with ideas. These talks about favorite events can often lead to joyful reminiscing on his part, so have your tape recorder handy.

Shopping

Dad easily gets overloaded and tired, so you keep your shopping simple. You've learned to adjust your pace to his and now you find yourself enjoying it. Little did you know that you'd take such pleasure in going to the hardware store, but now Dad gives you a tour with detailed explanations of the numerous bins of bolts, nails, and tools. He may be confused at home, but here in his element he has his old confidence back. It's his old stomping ground and you listen with delight to the man you used to know. There are days when you are the last "customers" to leave. It took visits to three different hardware stores before you found one with a staff and owner who encourage you to browse without spending a dime. Now several of the staff will take time to "talk shop" with Dad, and the owner gives Dad expired catalogs for his workshop at home.

◎

You and Mom have been going to the mall together for years, usually spending the better part of the day window shopping. Mom especially likes to browse at a couple of her favorite shops and then stop for lunch in the food court. These outings have always been fun for you both and you've reorganized your life to accomplish shopping for most clothes and other nonfood items on these trips. Mom takes special delight in helping you with your clothing selections, but occasionally she wants you to buy something that you definitely don't want. When at the register, you can replace it with your choice, but do it when she's not looking so her feelings don't get hurt. Letting Mom help choose your clothes seems to make it more acceptable to her when you make choices about her outfits.

◎

The local supermarket has wheelchairs with shopping baskets. As long as you don't need to do major shopping, the basket has sufficient room. You and Mom can fill the day, even if it's only to buy one particular item, like a box of bath salts or a basket of strawberries. After you get home you can talk about your experiences and some of the things you saw. She may not remember much about your outing, but it really doesn't matter. What's important is that she hears that you enjoyed her company and that you're pleased with her purchase. And on a positive note, the new bath salts may make bath time more enjoyable for her.

"We had a good time this morning when we went to the market. It'll be fun to try your new bath salts. I bet that apple scent is going to make a nice bath. I think we should try it out right now, don't you?"

While at the supermarket, go exploring something that's new to you: Greek stuffed grape leaves if you're Norwegian; Swedish meatballs if you're Indonesian. Or you and Mom can count the number of different brands of canned peas. You'll find that it doesn't really matter what you're looking at as long as you are sharing the experience.

(Also: Activities, Bath Time, Conversations, Crowds, Discussions, Identification, Projects, Personal Space, Safe Return, Walking)

Don't hurry, don't worry. You're only here for a short visit. So be sure to stop and smell the flowers.

-Walter C. Hagen

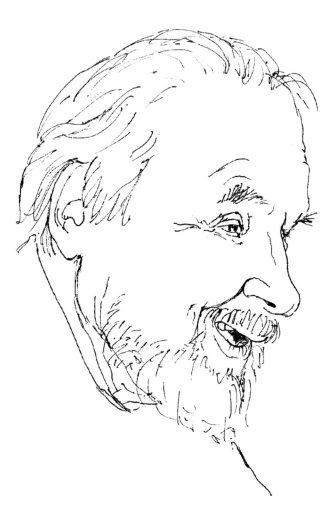

The great thing, and the hard thing, is to stick to things when you have outlived the first interest, and not yet got the second, which comes with a sort of mastery.
                                              -Janet Erskine Stuart

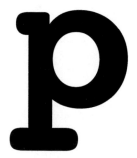

PACING

Dad has started pacing. He makes the rounds of your house by cruising down the hallway, through the kitchen down to the living room, and then back to the hall to start the cycle over again. It's distracting as well as distressing to you. You can usually guide him to his personal space, where you stay with him until he gets started on a project. He's very cooperative and stays for a few minutes, but then he resumes his rounds.

Pacing is not an uncommon behavior in Alzheimer's patients. When it occurs late in the day, it's known as sundowning. Dad may have an uncontrollable physical need to move, so you can help him by making sure that he has a safe path on which to pace, as well as plenty of liquids to drink so he doesn't get dehydrated.

Of course, his pacing may be psychological in nature. He may feel he's neglected to do something but he can't quite think of what it is, so he paces to try to remember or to calm down. This can be especially hard on him if he used to be an active person. He might need something mentally stimulating to help him focus. Consider setting up a workspace that relates to his career.

If he is on medication and his pacing is a sudden development, it's a good idea to talk to his doctor as soon as possible. Certain medications can cause physiological problems. Discuss with his doctor or pharmacist possible alternatives to the medication that might be causing him trouble.

(Also: Agitation, Diversions, Personal Space, Projects, Sundowning)

Success seems to be largely a matter of hanging on after others have let go.

-William Feather

PAIN

Mom has a nasty cut on the back of her hand and it's time to change the dressing and reapply ointment. It might be painful to Mom to remove the bandage, so soften it by applying warm water with a cotton ball. Carefully explain to her in your "coaching" voice what you're going to do:

"Mom, we have to change your bandage. You cut yourself and I have to put more ointment and a new one on it so it can heal again. Do you want to pull it off yourself? Or do you want me to do it?"

She may start to remove the bandage but she'll probably end up letting you do it in the end.

"I'll pull it off as gently as I can. I hope it won't hurt too much."

Mom will handle it best if you're honest with her, explaining everything that you're doing and why. She may need to hear you repeat it many times.

Because of her dementia, Mom sometimes forgets that she's got an injury or sore until it hurts her again. It's your natural inclination to comfort her if she feels a twinge in her bruised back and reacts with a whimper. With great solicitude in your voice you say,

"Oh, Mom, your back's hurting you again, isn't it?"

Unfortunately, while showing her that you're concerned, you have also unintentionally told her two things that she had completely forgotten because of her dementia: that her back is hurt and by the tone of your voice, that it must be serious.

You will help her more by maintaining a positive demeanor and not showing any worry in your voice. Instead, as she reacts to the twinge you say,

"Mom, let me help you sit up straight again so you can feel better."

Remember that because of her dementia, she has no recollection of her injury, so as soon as you make her more comfortable, she will forget about the pain.

(Also: Affections, Coaching, Diversions, Empathy, Humor)

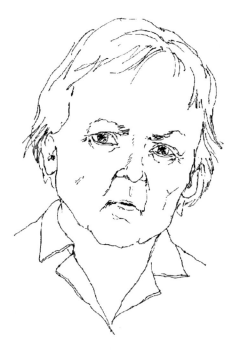

It takes courage to lead a life. Any life.
-Erica Jong

PAPER WORK

These personal papers should be with Mom at all times:

• One sheet of paper listing her social security number, Medicare, Medicaid, and other insurance information.
• List of emergency contact numbers
• Copy of the Durable Power of Attorney for Financial Matters
• Copy of Mom's Health Care Durable Power of Attorney
• Copy of Mom's DNR (Do Not Resuscitate) Order

DURABLE POWER OF ATTORNEY for Financial Matters is a notarized document that gives you the legal right to make financial and property decisions on your mother's behalf.

HEALTH CARE POWER OF ATTORNEY (HCPOA) is a signed document stating Mom's choices of the person(s)who will make health care choices for her if she's unable. This document usually includes provisions addressing the withdrawal of medical treatment if she has a terminal or incurable illness. (Also known as a Living Will.)

A DNR (Do Not Resuscitate) Order is a signed document stating that Mom does not want CPR in the event her heart stops. In instances where Mom's illness is significantly progressed, we strongly recommend that you establish a DNR Order for Mom and keep it with her at all times. CPR is rarely what we see on television or in the movies. In reality it's successful in only 5% of all attempts outside of the hospital. It can be extremely aggressive, often causing broken ribs and a crushed breastbone. Is this something you want Mom subjected to? Ask a local EMT, fire department, or hospital for a copy of their standard DNR order form. It's crucial that this document is instantly recognizable by any emergency personnel in your area if you want Mom's wishes to be respected.

Keep copies of Mom's HCPOA and DNR at all her doctors' offices, at her adult day-care center, and with any family members or friends with whom she spends time.

If Mom has started wandering, replicate the personal information sheet, add a recent 5x7 or 8x10 photograph (or photocopy of one) of Mom, and take them to your local police department. They can keep them on file in case they should find your Mom wandering. She should be wearing her medical alert identification bracelet at all times.

(Also: Identification, Neighborhood Flyer, Safe Return, Wandering)

The future comes one day at a time.
-Dean Acheson

PERSONAL SPACE

Before coming to live with you, Mom took great pride in her apartment and would spend hours cleaning and arranging her things. It was very hard on her to give it up and have to share a house with you. You've been doing your best to make her feel at home. Of course her own room is filled with her things, but you don't want her to spend her days squirreled away in her bedroom all day, so you've hung some of her pictures on the living-room walls and placed a few of her knickknacks among yours. One possible solution is to give her a daytime space of her own. It can be a whole room or just a corner of your workroom. The size of her "personal space" is less important than the feeling of this being her own domain. When you set aside an area specifically for her, you're letting her know that her interests are as important as your own. It helps give her a sense of purpose. Fill it with things relating to her favorite activities. Then when you need a diversion for her, you can steer her into this personal space and help her get started on a project.

Office

Dad ran his own company and retired a long time ago, but he's been quite confused lately, thinking he's still a working man. You've tried to convince him that he was lucky to be a retired man at leisure, but Dad is often miserable. He feels useless and gets angry. He frequently insists that he must go to the office. You try to tell him that he sold the business several years ago, but that only makes him more agitated.

One day you decide to go through some of his storage boxes in which you find some old company paperwork. It is a challenge for you to figure out which pieces of paper were "real" business documents to him, but you finally sort through them all. You make copies of the paperwork that will help you launch his new "office" in the corner of the kitchen where he keeps all his files, invoices, and notebooks.

Now, he'll spend hours with his work, sorting out papers and making copious notes in his date book. At the end of his "work day," whether it lasts thirty minutes or three hours, you try to make time for him and listen to his business plans and analysis. He can get on with the day, feeling a sense of accomplishment.

At one time in her life Mom had been a busy and successful buyer for a well-known women's clothing chain, so these days it's difficult for her to be idle. She often gets moody and restless in late afternoon, which was when she used to close the books at the end of the business day.

She needs to get back to "work," so you set up a desk for her in a corner of your home. Scout around the local office supply store for order forms, tally sheets, "in and out" baskets, a pencil caddy, paper clips, markers, high lighters, etc. Buy subscriptions to a couple of fashion magazines, get on the mailing lists of fashion catalogs, and collect fabric swatches.

Since she "goes to work" every afternoon with great determination, you're careful to respect her space:

"Excuse me, Mom, I'm sorry to interrupt. I'm making some coffee and I was wondering if you're ready for a break?"

At dinner, the two of you can share your day:

"How was your day? Did you get those orders done?"

You can browse boutiques together. You are impressed with her knowledge and clarity as you watch Mom scrutinizing styles, workmanship, and details. She may be very forgetful about other things, but she's quite lucid on these excursions. These times together are precious and it's a good idea to keep a journal of your experiences.

Studio

Mom fancied herself an artist when you were a child. She took classes in oil painting and watercolor techniques and she had a small easel set up in the corner of the laundry room. Although nothing ever became of it, her yearnings have never diminished.

Mom's been living with you for some time now. You go to galleries together and have had a lot of fun with collages and other craft projects. However, her dementia is getting worse and she's often agitated and restless. It helps her to create something. Set up projects that she can handle on her own without your participation, other than a word of encourage-ment now and then. You can set up a "studio" space her. Keep it small (a big studio can be too intimidating) with an easel, a canvas, and some basic supplies. On the other hand, she may no longer be able to create without your help, but since she's surrounded by items that remind her of the best of times, she may be happy arranging and rearranging her supplies. Ask your local art supply store for old cast-off stuff, like dried-up paint tubes.

You can also expand on Mom's projects by helping her do research on different artists or by maintaining files of art catalogs or scrapbooks with announcements, if she enjoys that sort of thing. Whenever she gets restless and needs a diversion, you can direct her to the studio. It's important that you treat her endeavors seriously.

In her personal "studio," you encourage Mom to talk about her work and you listen with sincerity. Don't gush over something she has created unless you mean it. She's likely to be aware if you're faking it. Instead ask her questions you know she can answer:

"I notice that you're using a lot of blue in your paintings. That's your favorite color, isn't it?"

Most of all, try to stay away from presuming that you know what it is she's painted. Don't say, "What's that supposed to be? A house?" unless you're absolutely sure that it really is a house. If Mom used to be a good artist but has now lost her painting skills, it might hurt her feelings to think that you can't recognize what she's painted.

Workshop

When you were a kid your Dad was always tinkering with one project or another in his beloved workshop. He had all kinds of tools then, although now you know he's not able to handle tools safely anymore.

Dad's been getting restless and has started pacing, so you set up a "shop" in the garage. Ask the local hardware store for some outdated catalogs and check out garage sales and flea markets for odds and ends in nuts, bolts, hooks, and other hardware items.

The next time Dad starts pacing, you can redirect him to his personal space:

"Did you find that tool you were looking for? What was it? A router?"

He disappears into his "shop" and returns a couple of minutes later with an armload of woodworking catalogs:

"No, of course not, I already have a router. Now where's that catalog? Come here, I'll show you."

You sit down with him and rifle through the catalogs together as he describes one tool after another. You find yourself caught up in his explanations and you ask questions in earnest. When he's talking "shop," he's the Dad you remember, knowledgeable and wise, with very little of his dementia in evidence.

(Also: Activities, Diversions, Exercise, Gardening, Kitchen, Outings)

If you are sure you understand everything that is going on, you are hopelessly confused.

-Walter Mondale

PETS

One day when you arrive early at the senior center to pick up Mom, you find her totally engrossed in a small dog brought by the local animal shelter volunteer. She's gently stroking the dog, a smile beaming on her face, making her look peaceful and happy. You'd once considered adopting a cat or a dog, but were concerned that it would be too much for Mom. Watching her enjoyment has made you reconsider the possibility.

It has long been recognized that animals have a positive therapeutic effect. Just stroking a dog or a cat can lower the stress level and blood pressure. More progressive nursing homes are even employing furry "pet therapists," because of their soothing effects on the residents. Cats, dogs, and rabbits are favorites.

You can contact your local shelter and ask them to keep an eye out for a sweet and gentle cat or dog for Mom. Puppies and kittens are adorable, but they are frisky and may be harder for Mom to handle, so it's probably a better idea to get an adult pet.

If your landlord does not permit pets, consider setting up a fish tank. It's very soothing and calming just to watch the fish swim by. Some educational toy stores sell a fake aquarium that is so realistic that Mom may attempt to feed the fish.

(Also: Affections)

The greatest pleasure of a dog is that you may make a fool of yourself with him, and not only will he not scold you, but he will make a fool of himself, too.

-Samuel Butler

PILLS

Mom needs to take her supplements. As you hand her the first tablet and a glass of water or juice, explain to her what these supplements are and how they benefit her:

"These are your vitamins, Mom. I've noticed a real improvement in your health since you've been taking them. Now, here's the first one: it's easy to swallow. Then take sip of juice and swallow everything."

Give her each tablet with the same thorough explanation, if it's necessary. Remember that tomorrow you'll go through the same routine all over again.

If Mom can't swallow her pills, try crushing them and mixing them with something tasty like chocolate frosting, applesauce, jam, or even ranch dressing. You might want to taste each one of her supplements to find food or drink that could disguise a foul tasting pill. Some medications, such as B-Complex vitamins, can't be disguised no matter what you do, though some sublingual vitamin Bs come in a fruit flavor.

Be honest with her when you present her with a teaspoon of the unusual mixture:

"Mom, I've mixed your pill with some jelly. It still tastes a little weird, but it's not too bad."

If you continue to have problems, even with crushed pills, ask your pharmacist for liquid versions. Many painkillers, cold remedies, and multivitamins are available in liquid form.

(Also: Coaching, Honesty, Medications)

PRIVACY

Dad lives in your spare bedroom now. He's surrounded by his personal belongings and you have a sign on his door with either his name or "Dad" on it, whichever he prefers. You respect his privacy and treat his room as his own domain, always knocking before entering, even if you leave his door ajar so you can keep an eye on him.

Knock, knock:
"Excuse me, Dad, may I come in? I would like to make your bed. Is now a good time?"

Knock, knock:
"Good morning, Dad. May I come in so I can help you get dressed and then we'll eat breakfast."

Knock, knock.
"Excuse me, Dad, may I come in?"

"NO!"

"Oh, I'm sorry, I didn't realize you were busy. I'll come back later. Will ten minutes be good?"

"Okay."

One common anxiety among Alzheimer's folks is the loss of self-determination. By respecting his private space, you help Dad maintain a feeling of control of his space and his life. Even if he's bedridden you want to continue to knock before entering.

(Also: Dignity, Environment, Independence)

PROJECTS

Retirement can be difficult for Dad. He no longer has his job to give him a reason to get up in the morning, the validation in the form of a paycheck. Successful retirees find substitute activities to keep themselves stimulated and vital. Because of his dementia, Dad's not able to do this for himself. He needs you to help make things happen for him. We give you many ideas in three different areas: Games and stimulating group projects, excursions, and special activity rooms or areas at home. Initially it may take some extra effort on your part, but the payoff will be a happier Dad and an easier life for both of you.

The success of Dad's projects will hinge more than anything on your attitude. No matter what activity he gets involved in, it's important that you take it seriously. However simple or uncomplicated the project might be, your reaction will give it validity and importance.

Dad has been restless since breakfast. He needs something to do to help him get back to feeling good about himself. You begin by asking for his help:

"Excuse me, Dad, are you busy right now? I sure could use your help. Let me show you. You see this stack of catalogs? I can't make heads or tails of them. Could you help me sort them out, please?... (After he agrees:) Let's see: we have wood-working, computer stuff, linens, and outdoor clothes. How do you suggest we do it?"

Wait for his suggestion and no matter what it is, let him know you think it's a good one. It's important that you not talk to him like a child; he's demented but he's not stupid.

Art Projects

You and Mom can create art out of anything, from string and fabric to old toothbrushes. You can paste things onto cardboard, mount them in boxes, or make freestanding sculptures. Remember, there are no rules on what is or isn't art!

Ideas:

• Cardboard milk cartons make wonderful "shrines." You can cutout the front panel or divide it into two folding door panels and spray paint it gold, silver, or any color of your choice. Then you can place an arrangement of little items you've collected inside your shrine, i.e. pine cones, tiny thumb-sized dolls, broken brooches, pebbles, leaves. You can paint them or leave them in their natural state. It's entirely up to you!

• Flower pots, baskets, or picture frames all make good starts for your art pieces. You can decorate them with ribbons and odd buttons, paint them, decoupage them with magazine pictures, or cover them with pasta shapes and spray paint.

• Found objects can become "sculptures," things from nature like leaves, twigs, cones, and nuts. Also wood scraps, hardware, broken tools, nuts, bolts, old kitchen tools, old flatware, broken dishes, pottery shards, pieces of tile, party favors, small toys, watch parts, and old jewelry. You can mount your objects with white glue, contact cement, Liquid Nails, or set them in tile-setting cement.

Collages

You discovered making collages by accident. You'd run out of gift wrap while wrapping a birthday present, so you used plain tissue paper and then you'd cut out a bunch of colorful pictures from old magazines and pasted them all over the tissue. Your wrapping paper was the hit of the party. You had so much fun that you decided to try it again, this time on poster board. Since then you've collected a big box full of all sorts of images for your collages.

Since Mom loves animals, you collect old National Geographic magazines, and nature calendars. To help Mom make a no-fail collage, you start by covering the board with colored paper, construction paper, or calendar pictures. Mom can cut out pictures, using safety scissors if necessary, but she may have trouble handling the glue stick, so you help her paste the cutouts in an overlapping manner. You'll get the best results if you avoid cutting straight edges. Here are some ideas:

• A big tree collage composed of images from a nature calendar? You can use tiny cutout pictures of birds and paste them all over the "branches" of the collage trees.

• A collage of desserts from food or home magazines?

• A glamour collage: Start with a large picture of a woman's face and surround her with lots of tiny overlapping cutouts, so that at a distance they look like cascading hair.

As you gain creative confidence, you can make a collage of images of your family. Have copies made of all the photos, so you don't have to cut up the originals.

Crafts

Mom would often relax with her knitting or crochet when you were a kid. Recently you discover her old needles and some yarns. You eagerly bring them to her, but she only fiddles with them for a while and then sets them aside, seemingly having forgotten what to do with them.

Remembering how much she had enjoyed creating something, you search for something more appropriate. You find books on crafts projects and buy all the supplies you need: felt squares, foam balls, glue, and safe scissors. You set it up in front of her with great expectations, but again she just stares at the pile of art supplies. Nothing you say inspires her.

"Mom, see what I got for you? You can make a lovely gift . . Cut this out . . . now this . . . fold this and glue this on . . ." etc.

"Well, why don't you make it, if it's supposed to be so lovely?" She replies tartly.

Ah ha! You decide to participate. You pull up a chair and start working on the project with her. You follow the directions closely. Halfway through, you're totally confused. Your project looks nothing like the picture in the directions.

"Mom, this doesn't look right. What do you think we should do with it now?"

You have reached a crossroads at this point; you either scrap the whole thing or go hog wild with what you've already created. You grab the first thing in front of you, cut it up, and glue it on. You throw in some glitter, pieces of yarn or ribbon. After a while Mom joins in. It's just too irresistible.

Whatever your end result, you've both had a great time and you've discovered the secret to your success: working together, remembering there are no rules when it comes to creativity, and having no expectations of perfect results. The most important thing is that you had fun. Together!

Fiddle Boxes

Dad likes to keep things organized. He helps you sort out the mail and painstakingly stacks magazines by titles and dates. These tasks have been successful diversions for him. You can expand on this idea by creating "fiddle boxes." Use an assortment of old cartons or shoeboxes and load them with interesting items that lend themselves to categorizing, sorting, or counting. One box can be stocked with screws, nails, washers, and other hardware trinkets. Another has a collection of odd buttons. Fiddle boxes can hold fabric scraps, cookie cutters, old postcards, old jewelry, or other smallish items. You keep fiddle boxes close at hand when you need them as diversions for Dad when he's restless:

"Dad, I really could use some help. I found this box. Look at it, it's a godawful mess. I'm just too busy right now to clean it up. Could you spare a few minutes to help me out? Who knows what interesting stuff you'll find in all this mess."

It's important that you treat these fiddle boxes as serious projects and you're careful not to let on to him that you've created them especially as diversions for him. After he has "helped" you, you'll want to spend a few minutes admiring his handiwork and be sure to thank him for his hard work.

Jigsaw Puzzles

Years ago Mom was a whiz with those big 1,000-piece puzzles that would take several days to finish, but now she has trouble coping with ones that have only 50 pieces. You'd like to buy her jigsaw puzzles with just a few pieces, but those are usually designed for children.

Consider making your own puzzles. The number of pieces should be determined by Mom's ability, so start with puzzles of ten big pieces.

How To:

Supplies: Foam core, spray adhesive, a size 11 X-acto knife, and pages from a calendar, a full-page image from a magazine, or an 8 1/2" x 11" color copy of a family picture.

Have Mom select the image. Spray the back of the picture with spray adhesive and paste it on a piece of foam core that is the same size as the picture. Let it dry and then cut it with the X-acto knife into no more than ten puzzle pieces. Don't worry about cutting intricate tabs or shapes; stick with uncomplicated curves.

Painting

Someone suggested that you try getting Dad to paint as a form of therapy. Who? Your Dad? The man who always thought that artists were a bunch of weirdoes? But you need something entertaining for him to do and you know he likes to do things with his hands, so why not try?

As with any new activity that you introduce to Dad, you join in with him. You're a novice at this art stuff too, so it becomes a new adventure for both of you.

You're going to experiment and mess around, so you don't want to buy expensive canvases or watercolor paper that imply expectations of "serious" work. Instead go to your local frame shop for mat board and foam core remnants or to a variety store for poster board. Visit your local builders' supply or hobby shop for inexpensive bristle and foam brushes, 1/2" to 3" wide. Lastly, buy a few bottles of inexpensive waterbased poster paints.

Protect your largest indoor or outdoor table by covering it with newsprint or a dropcloth. Lay out a single piece of posterboard or a piece of mat board so that you can both work together on one painting. Most importantly, don't take this seriously! Use wide brushes to keep yourself from getting stuck on details, and remember that abstract painting is perfectly acceptable! The point of this project is to have fun, not to produce a Rembrandt-like masterpiece. What makes this a wonderful activity is the process of creating and experimenting together. You may not make serious art but you're guaranteed to make serious fun.

Wetting down the board gives the effect of watercolor and will aid in your colors flowing together. Dip your brush in a bright color and make a large stroke across the entire surface. Invite Dad to dip his brush in a different color and make his sweeping stroke. Repeat this a few times and pretty soon you'll have either a mud-colored mess or an interesting "abstract" painting.

"Not bad! Look at these colors and shapes. I didn't know we were such good artists, did you? Let's paint another one or would you like to paint on your own?" He's likely to need several joint sessions with you before he's secure enough to work by himself.

Scrapbooks
Mom's especially fond of animals and you keep a scrapbook for her in which she collects pictures cut from nature and pet magazines. Every so often you'll both sit down and look for new images.

"Mom, you said you'd like to work on your animal book. Would you mind if I helped you?"

Mom likes to arrange her pictures. You help her write down on each page classifications, such as species, home countries, color, or size.

Make sure that she has a wide variety of pictures to sort through. You'll find that Mom will become totally engrossed in these projects, as long as you treat them seriously.

Dad has a passion for sports cars. For years he'd pile up automobile magazines in the garage. You've found that he'll spend time contemplating pictures of car designs since you've encouraged him to keep a scrapbook of his very favorites.

You can collect images of just about anything to make a scrapbook, from babies to furniture, from flowers to recipes.

(Also: Activities, Choices, Coaching, Dignity, Empathy, Outings, Personal Space)

It is good to have an end to journey towards;
but it is the journey that matters in the end.
-Ursula K. LeGuin

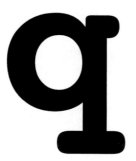

QUESTIONS

Your communication with Mom has improved immensely since you've followed our ideas. Still you often find yourself in a bind when you ask Mom questions and don't get the responses you were expecting. Try asking questions in a way that does not trigger immediate resistance from Mom. Try to phrase your questions so you'll get the response you desire. Instead of saying,

"Do you want to take your vitamins?"

To which you may get a resounding: "No!"

Try this approach:

"Before you eat your eggs, let me give you vitamins. Here, let's take this one first. It's the one that's good for your heart. Here you are, open up your mouth wide. (Open your own mouth wide and she'll likely mimic you.) There you are! You did it! Thank you. Now you're ready for your eggs."

Mom may not remember from one day to the next what you're talking about, so preface your questions with a short recap:

"Yesterday we bought these pads for you to wear at night. Then if you have a small accident you won't have to worry about it. You thought it was a good idea. You can put one on now, before you put on your pajamas. That sounds like a good plan, doesn't it?"

You'll want to phrase your questions so the natural answer is what you want. Just think of it: If you say, "You don't want to do this, do you?" saying "No" would be the natural response, but if you say, "You want to do this, don't you?" you'll more likely get a "Yes." Also, if you nod your head at the same time you'll elicit a positive response most of the time.

Any question that presses Mom's memory may upset her, so you want to be very careful with anything having to do with recall. Drop from your vocabulary phrases like: "Do you remember?" "Don't you remember?" and "Have you forgotten?"

Mom may recall if given an introduction by you in the way of a recap or overview. It'll take some practice to get into the habit of detailed explanations, but after a while it'll be second nature to you, Mom will feel more secure, and you'll get results where you used to feel frustrated. The bonus for Mom is the focus she senses from you.

(Also: Choices, Coaching, Communication, Listening, No!, Normal)

It's better to know some of the questions than all of the answers.
                             -James Thurber

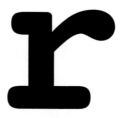

REACTIONS

As soon as you think you have things under control, something happens that catches you so off guard that it's all you can do not to react.

Mom's waiting in the car while you go to post a letter. In the two minutes you're gone, she has somehow managed to remove her blouse. It wouldn't be so bad except for the fact that she's not wearing anything else underneath. The parking lot is crowded with people while your mother's sitting half naked in full view. You're mortified and want to scream at her. You want to disown her or put her in a nursing home first thing in the morning!

Instead, take at least two deep breaths so you can get into the car with Mom calmly. Open the window to cool her off and help her put on her blouse:

"It sure got hot, didn't it? I'll open this window and then I'll help you put your blouse back on. I think we should find a place to have a glass of lemonade. What do you say?"

Mom does not mean to upset you. In her confusion, she may not be able to think past her most immediate concern, which in this case is to cool herself off. She probably isn't aware that she's in the car. If you had scolded her, she'd only become embarrassed about something that has already happened and cannot be changed. Because of her memory problems, it's likely she wouldn't be able to connect your reaction to her removing her blouse in public.

◎

You hear a buzzing noise coming from the garage and, realizing that Dad is no longer in his easy chair, you dash out there. Dad is at your workbench with your portable saw and a very small piece of wood. A sure recipe for disaster! He is about to start cutting when you enter. Your instinct is to scream at him to halt, but you realize in that moment that your outburst might startle and cause him to cut himself. Hard as it is, you've learned to hold your reactions and stay relatively calm. You quickly go to his side.

"Dad, may I interrupt you? I would like very much to watch you. You are so knowledgeable and I always learn something from you. What d'you say we eat first? Lunch is ready and you look hungry. Then later this afternoon we can look at your plans together."

You have avoided a potential disaster with a diversion and you have paid him a compliment by showing that you are interested in his projects.

(Also: Coaching, Communication, Dignity, Empathy, No!, Normal, Personal Space, Projects)

READING

Mom was once an avid reader who'd been very proud of her book collection. You've set up a special reading corner for her in your apartment with a bookshelf filled with her favorite titles. She still loves to hold a book while sitting in her big, comfy chair beside the reading lamp. She rarely gets beyond the first page, but she's still happy as a clam. The two of you can spend hours sharing your quiet reading time as you read your book and she "reads" hers.

There are other times when you'll want to enhance your shared experience by reading out loud to her. Anything can be interesting to her when you read it with enthusiasm. Try reading a "good news" item in the daily paper, though upbeat articles can be scarce. Or you might read a cookbook out loud and fantasize about a huge dinner with rich desserts and then laugh about not having gained an ounce. Gourmet, Bon Appetit, or Saveur magazines have especially delectable descriptions of meals.

If Mom has a special interest in something specific, such as archaeology or history, then consider taking a trip to the local library in order to find books on the subject. Mom will enjoy discovering them and it'll be a pleasure for her to hear them read out loud. When she shows special interest in a book, you can check it out to share later.

(Also: Discussions, Outings)

Stories are medicine ... They have such power; they do not require that we do, be, act anything ----we need only listen.
                              -Clarissa Pinkola Estes, Ph.

REALITY

You and your wife have such a close relationship that it never crossed your mind that things would ever be anything different. Now you realize that although she looks and sounds like your wife, the person you knew is no longer living inside that body. You keep searching for her, feeling sad and angry that she's no longer there. You think that if only you could remind her of who she is, then surely she'd snap out of it. You want to shake the "real" person out of her. Many of us have the mistaken assumption that if we insist on reminding her that her reality is wrong, crazy, or misguided, then she'll remember and everything will be fine again, the way it once was. But it will never be the way it used to be. You'll only succeed in causing both of you needless anguish by trying to force her to look at a reality that she can no longer grasp. The most beneficial thing that you can do is to get to know and accept the new person that she has become.

Your wife rarely remembers in the usual sense of the word. What often happens is that she relives rather than remembers her experiences, there being a very important distinction between the two. She is completely in the "here and now" of a particular memory, as if it were happening all over again. You can increase the chances of success with your wife if you try to live in the "here and now" with her too. Take each moment for what it is at that particular time.

She seems to escape more and more into her memories, but then, who can blame her? After all, the present can be so confusing. Sometimes she can't remember things that just happened, yet she can often relive an event from thirty, even sixty, years ago.

"Mother's making lunch and I have to go home right now or she'll be mad at me," your wife says.

She's reliving a moment in time when she was a child. Try to refrain from forcing the reality of the moment on her with remarks like:

"You live here! In this house! With me! And your mother died a long time ago!"

Knowing that this flashback feels totally real to her, join her there in the relived experience. Put your arm around her and say,

"Your mother called and said she'll be here later, so she wants us to go ahead and eat dinner."

Or: "Why don't we call her and invite her to come here to visit us tomorrow?"

On the other hand, your wife may still be aware on some level that her mother is no longer alive. In that case, be very gentle with her and explain:

"Sweetheart, your mother's been gone for several years now. It's still hard for me to believe. Sometimes I pick up the phone to call her before I remember that she's no longer with us. But I am so glad that we have each other. You know, sweetie, dinner is almost ready and you know that your dear mother would have been pretty upset if we let it go to waste. While we're getting everything ready, you can tell me more about your mother's cooking. The other day you were talking about her great mashed potatoes. We can make some tomorrow, okay? Would you help me set the table, please?"

This approach allows you to return the conversation back to the present in a much gentler manner.

You're cooking dinner when Dad comes stomping into the kitchen wearing big rubber boots and a rain slicker. He's furious that Larry is late:

"Where the heck is that guy? He knows we need to get out to the lake by dusk. Larry's never on time for anything. I don't know why I bother..."

Dad and Larry were best buddies as teenagers and fishing was one of their shared passions. There's no point in arguing with him that this is "here and now" and that he's eighty something and hasn't seen Larry in sixty years. At this particular time he's eighteen years old again. What would calm him down at this moment? You can use a loving lie followed by a diversion.

"Larry called and said he'll meet you when we're done eating. Let me hang up your raincoat until you're ready to go. It's too uncomfortable to wear that at the table, isn't it? . . . By the way Dad, you were going to tell me about that weird tool we saw yesterday at the hardware store. You said it was some kind of saw."

Soon he's forgotten all about the fishing trip.

(Also: Empathy, Loving Lies, Normal)

Since we cannot change reality,
let us change the eyes which see reality.
-Nikos Kazantzakis

RECORDING MEMORIES

There might be times when you wish that you had a camera permanently aimed at Dad. Only then could you capture one of those precious moments when he comes out with a funny-sweet remark that might lose some of its charm if you tried to write it down in your journal.

If you have a camcorder, set up the camera on a high surface or a tripod and just let it run for an afternoon. It may sound uninteresting now, but later on you will probably appreciate these tapes because they are the irreplaceable memories of your real life with Dad.

There are so many events, great and small, that you'll want to preserve for yourself and for the family archives. They can be funny, sweet, or bizarre stories, or the occasions when Dad gets on a roll and starts to reminisce. Even if you've heard his stories a hundred times before, try to record them for the rest of your family. They are a part of your life's history, whether or not they're even true. The videos you record of Dad telling stories will be treasures in years to come.

You can also keep a small cassette audio recorder in your purse or pocket so you can record what Dad has to say anytime, anywhere. You can also use the recorder to take verbal notes that you can later transcribe into your journal.

(Also: Journals, Memories, Questions)

Recall it as often as you wish,
a happy memory never wears out.
-Libbie Fudim

REPETITIONS

Dad tells a handful of old stories so often that you know them all by heart, yet he has trouble remembering the simplest things like where the bathroom is or how to hold a fork. It's helpful to put up signs to direct him to the bathroom and you can place the fork in his hand as you direct it gently to his mouth.

You patiently talk him through the motions:

"Here's your fork, Dad. You hold it in this hand, then pick up a bite of food and then you bring it to your mouth."

Hopefully he remembers this by the next bite, but chances are you'll have to repeat these directions several times during the meal.

It's hard not to be impatient with Dad with this continuous repetition and a few times you've slipped and blurted out,

"But I just showed you!"

Unfortunately, you've just reminded him of his problem. It's likely that Dad responds with increased confusion. You need to help him calm down again. You can offer to warm his food, add some more gravy, or offer him a pickle. Any of these diversions may get him refocused and give you a chance to start over again.

Now, that you've lived with Dad's dementia for awhile, you're becoming accustomed to repeating your directions calmly as often as you feel it is necessary:

"The bathroom's down the hallway. Do you see the sign on the wall? Just follow the signs, Dad. Let me know if you'd like me to show you."

Listen carefully to make sure he gets there all right. If not, catch up to him and redirect him with a cheerful,

"Here's a sign that says "Bathroom." We follow the arrows. Here's another sign. Here we are!"

Mom's trying to put on her shoes. She can't quite figure out how to position her foot, so you guide it into the first shoe, while you explain to her,

"We'll put the shoe here in front of you, then you can slide your toes inside and then the rest of your foot. Just like that! You've got it!"

Now you repeat the exact same directions with the second shoe. This repetition used to be maddening, but now you're used to coaching her through dressing, eating, bathing, walking, and other actions that may bewilder her. Your cheerful attitude keeps her feeling cooperative and secure. After particularly confusing times when it's clear to you that she's trying really hard, it's so natural for you to respond to her with a big hug.

(Also: Coaching, Communication, Questions)

Unselfish and noble actions are the most radiant pages in the biography of souls.

-David Thomas

RESPITE

You and Dad get along well from day to day. You've set up his personal space, which keeps him happily occupied while giving you a little time for yourself. You've gotten pretty good at communicating with him, even as he's losing his speech. You've put up signs all over the house to help him function on his own. Everything seems fine, but there are still times when you feel trapped by your situation and you feel guilty and ashamed that you feel that way. You need some relief!

Taking care of a person with Alzheimer's is a major undertaking that should be shared, and you have the right to insist that family pitch in. Arrange for your siblings or family members to stay with Dad at your house for long weekends or have Dad spend time at their homes so that you can take a break. This will not only give you the time off you deserve, it will also give them the chance to participate in caring for Dad so they can see for themselves how he's really doing.

You may have a fulltime job and be the sole caregiver for Dad. This probably leaves you with little or no private time.

Take advantage of all the local support that is available to you: the Alzheimer's Association holds support group meetings in most communities, and other government agencies, like your local Ombudsman's office, can direct you to local programs that can give both you and Dad a respite.

With any luck, your city has an adult day-care center where Dad can spend a few hours several days a week. You can also ask your local Alzheimer's Association or senior center to help you make contact with one or two other families in order to create a "share-care" group. Sharing outings with your group are more fun and easier on individual caregivers. You can also take turns caring for all your elders for a day. Though you may find it hard work looking after more than one elder at a time, it'll be well worth it. When it's your turn to take a day off, you can blissfully enjoy it, knowing that Dad's in a safe and loving environment where he's being cared for by people familiar to him.

Your "share-care" group can also take turns relieving each other in the evenings. You're all entitled to a periodic night out, dinners with friends, theater, movies, or a massage.

When you feel refreshed and invigorated you can approach your caregiving tasks with new energy. Dad will reflect how you feel in his mood and behavior.

(Also: Day Care, Family, Home Help, Share-Care, Support Groups)

Work is not always required ...
there is such a thing as sacred idleness,
the cultivation of which is now fearfully neglected.
-George Macdonald

RESTAURANTS

Going out to eat is a special event for Mom. She'll look intently at the menu, often upside down. She remembers the concept of reading, but she's not exactly sure how to do it anymore. Let her hold the menu any way she wants, while you read out loud from your own menu. You can point out her favorite dish:

"Look Mom, they have your favorite dish. Would you like to have that today, or would you like to try something new?"

No matter how she responds, you can order something you know she'll be able to eat without too many difficulties and when it comes to your table you present it to her with a big smile.

"Here it is, just what you ordered. It sure looks delicious."

She may get confused if there are too many different kinds of foods on her plate, or if she's given too many utensils at one time. Ask the waiter to bring an extra plate so you can separate fork food from finger food and serve her one kind at a time. Give her one utensil, either a fork or spoon, whichever is appropriate for the dish. It's important for her dignity that she continues to use the appropriate utensils for as long as possible. She may not be able to handle a knife efficiently or safely, so you can either choose something that doesn't need cutting or cut it up for her in advance.

※

Mom wants a sandwich, but her hands have forgotten how to hold it. Either you can cut it up so that Mom can eat it with a fork, or ask the waiter to bring the contents of her sandwich, without the bread, so she can eat it with a fork. If it comes with finger food like chips or fries, put them on a separate plate for her to eat after she's finished her fork food.

Try to allot plenty of time for lunch and let Mom set the pace. You may want to frequent cafeterias or buffet restaurants where the waiters aren't dependent on tips and turnover. That way you can take your time and linger over your meal. It's important, however, occasionally to eat at restaurants because the experience can make Mom feel elegant and special. Consider going to restaurants during off-hours, either before or after the crowds.

On your ride home, you can talk to her about how nice the meal was and she can help you make plans for a return visit. You can reiterate with her what you had both enjoyed. You can compare and discuss the ingredients. Talking about your meals in such minute details helps Mom stay with the immediate memory. You're also reiterating how much you enjoyed sharing this experience with her. Restaurants make great conversation topics, because food is something we can all discuss and we usually have strong opinions and likes and dislikes.

(Also: Coaching, Crowds, Dignity, Eating)

Keep breathing.
-Sophie Tucker

ROUTINES

Mom grew up in a family that followed strict routines. Even though she has dementia, she still likes to do things in a certain way and at a certain time. She's reassured by the familiarity of habit. She'll set the table for you, always laying out the silverware just so, the napkins absolutely perpendicular, and her chair always facing a certain direction at the table. Almost every day she'll insist that dinner should be on time. Your personal lifestyle is usually much more relaxed, so it can be annoying when she gets so controlling and inflexible.

Following routines can be very important to folks with dementia, however. It gives them a sense of anchoring if they know when it's time to bathe, put on shoes, or eat. You're learning to adjust to life by the clock, much to Mom's relief. When Mom is happy, life is a lot easier for the both of you. You have learned to take advantage of her near-obsessive thinking by posting a couple of big signs noting her weekly bath time. What used to be a major battle has become relatively easy now, because if Mom resists bathing, you can simply point to the sign in the bathroom:

"Well, let's see, here it says: Bath time – Wednesday at 2 p.m. Well, today is Wednesday and my watch says two o'clock. How about yours? I'll be glad to give you a hand. I'll start the water while you choose the soap."

You can have signs in the bathroom: Mom's soap, Mom's towel, Mom's bath time: Wednesdays. This will help maintain your bath routines.

(Also: Bathroom, Coaching, Eating)

RUNNING COMMENTARY

You're getting used to talking your way through most of the things you do with or around Mom. It was awkward at first, making you feel kind of silly to think out loud like that, but now this new skill helps you to coach Mom when necessary:

"Let me see, I'm going to clear these dishes and take them to the kitchen and wash them . . . Look at this: This is one of the glasses you gave me. I'm going to carry it out by itself. I have to be really careful with it, so it doesn't break . . . and now we'll write our grocery list. Maybe we'll have spaghetti tonight? Nah, we just had that two days ago. Let me think . . . how about chicken? We have that new chicken recipe we wanted to try. I wonder if we have enough onions and garlic . . . Oh, I guess it doesn't matter, one can never have too many onions, so we might as well get some more . . . and some mushrooms, and oh, of course: ice cream! I almost forgot (ha, ha.) You'd never speak to me again if I forgot the ice cream, would you?"

Ask for Mom's opinion often, even if she's not coherent or her "input" has no relation to your question. Simply respond as if she's offered an excellent idea, but don't go overboard in your positive reaction. Keep it natural and sincere.

@

As tedious as this rambling chitchat might seem, it helps Dad by getting him used to hearing you "talk through directions" which will be beneficial in situations when you need to get him to do things he's reluctant to do:

"I have to pay a bunch of bills. Do you want to keep me company? Let me see. What do we have here? This one is from the Phone Company. Wow, look at these long distance charges. I think we should look into changing to another company. What do you think? . . . You know, nowadays we can choose our long distance company, not like the old days when there was only one. Now there are so many it's totally confusing. Now, look at this bill. This is not bad. I thought our electric bill would've been higher, because we sure watched a lot of television last week. We watched that great show about the gorillas that use sign language. We made a video copy of that so we can watch it again any time we want. Isn't that great? Would you like to watch it later? – Oh, darn! My pen just ran out of ink. There must be another pen in this drawer. Let me see. Well, I see a fat marker and a stumpy pencil. I can't very well write a check with either one, can I? Do you have a pen in your pocket, Dad? No? Okay, I guess I'll have to get up and go look in the desk in the living room. Don't go away. I'll be right back.". . . etc.

৵❧

You and Mom have gone shopping at a local discount store. The place is so cavernous that you gladly take advantage of their courtesy wheelchairs. Mom's having a hard time concentrating on regular conversation, so you use your "running commentary" to help her feel connected:

"Let's see, we need to find a dishpan. Now where would you go, Mom? How about the kitchen department? I'd think so, after all, that's where you'd wash dishes, right? I mean in the kitchen, not in the kitchen department! . . . OK, here we are! Now I see pots and pans. I see apple peelers, tomato slicers, carrot graters, ice cream scoops, butter scoops, soup scoops. Oh, that's right, they're called ladles, aren't they? . . . Do you see a dishpan, Mom? Do I see a dishpan? Of course not. That would've been too easy. So, now we start over again. Let's look at the signs: Shoes, Automotive, Furniture, Toys . . . I don't know, I don't see a sign that says dishpans, do you? Do you feel up to going up and down the aisles until we find it? Good, they've gotta have a dishpan and we need a dishpan! Let's go up through this aisle . . . Here we have some really weird-looking picture frames and look at those lamps. They have some kind of oil in them. Have you ever seen anything like that? Me neither. Oh, look, there's a bucket and a rack of brooms and what do you know – dishpans! Hallelujah! Let's pay for it and get on home. What do you say?"

As you're roaming through the store, take time to look at interesting stuff along the way. By the time you get home, it will have felt enough like a major excursion that it'll keep the two of you talking about it well into the evening.

(Also: Communication, Comprehension, Outings)

Life is not a static thing. The only people who do not change their minds are incompetents in asylums, and those in cemeteries.

-Everett McKinley

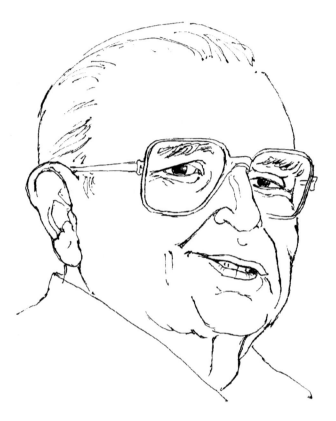

To be really great in little things, to be truly noble and
heroic in the insipid details of everyday life, is a virtue so
rare as to be worthy of canonization.
                                        -Harriet Beecher Stowe.

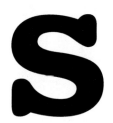

SAFE RETURN

Sponsored by the Alzheimer's Association, the Safe Return program assists in the safe and timely return of a person with Alzheimer's disease or dementia who wanders. It works very simply: When you register, for a modest fee, you are supplied with an identification bracelet or necklace engraved with:

"Memory Impaired.
To help (Dad's name) call 1(800) 572-1122, ID #"

If Dad wanders off, anyone who encounters him can call the hotline 24 hours a day. The hotline will then contact you with his location. Likewise, you can call the hotline to alert them when Dad's gone missing. The program maintains a national database that includes important emergency contact information and photographs to help unite lost individuals with their caregivers, no matter where they may wander.

Contact Safe Return at (888) 572-8566
or call the Alzheimer's Association at (888) 572-3900.

(Also: Identification, Neighborhood Flyer, Wandering)

SEXUALITY

Mom's been going to the monthly socials at the senior center. You drop her off and knowing that she's in a safe place, you can treat yourself to a couple of much needed hours of respite. She loves dancing to the oldies. Lately, she's had a steady dance partner and they have such a good time that you invite him for dinner at your house. He lives alone and reciprocates. Before long they're seeing each other quite frequently. You'll drive her to his place and occasionally drop them off at a restaurant or movie theater.

One day you arrive early to pick Mom up and you find the two of them locked in a passionate embrace. You're shocked. It had never occurred to you that there would be anything physical between them. Sure, you'd read many articles about sex in old age, but you never thought of Mom in those terms. Truth be told, you never thought of her as a sexual being, even when she was young. Few of us think of our parents that way.

When you've had a chance to calm down, you realize just how lucky Mom is. This lovely man is obviously fond of her and accepts her, dementia and all, so you're going to do all you can to support their relationship. From now on you're careful to arrive on time and when he visits at your house, you respect their privacy in her room.

Mom's friend often acts as an interpreter for her with you and the outside world. He is one person who truly knows what you're dealing with and with whom you can discuss difficult situations. He could become your strongest ally.

ॐ

Your Dad and Mom have both been living with you, because of Mom's severe dementia. They still have an active sex life. One evening you hear a blood curdling scream from their bedroom.

"Don't touch me! Get this man out of my room! Who are you? Get away from me!"

Dad comes flying out of the room, half-naked and near tears.

"Your Mother threw the phone at me. She doesn't know who I am. Oh my, what am I gonna do?"

You quickly give Dad a hug and dash to Mom's side to calm her down. She's oblivious to what has just happened.

You've never had to talk to Dad about their private life before, but now you're thrown right in the middle of it. Invite him to talk about his feelings and let him know that you understand his distress. If he's comfortable with the idea, suggest to him that he limit himself to affectionate stroking, hugging, holding, and touching, so your Mom will be less likely to freak out. Encourage him to talk to the support group and offer to go along with him for emotional support, since he might not feel entirely comfortable with discussing his situation with a group. After all, he belongs to a generation that believed in keeping one's feelings private, especially if you were a man.

Delicate Situations

It's a beautiful morning. You have a wonderful day planned so you're feeling great when you go to wake up Mom. You knock on her door and she doesn't answer, which isn't unusual, so you walk in. You stop dead in your tracks when you realize that Mom is contentedly playing with herself. She doesn't see you, so you make a fast exit. You know that masturbation is a perfectly natural activity, but Mother? For a moment you're gasping for air. How are you going to deal with this? You know that Mom would positively die of embarrassment if she knew that you'd seen her.

Shaken, you take a deep breath as you retreat to the kitchen to calm down. There really isn't anything you can do about it, other than make sure that from now on you're not so quick to enter her room. You'll probably look at Mom with different eyes now, realizing that she's still a woman with normal urges, just like you. It may take you a while to adjust, but as you become more comfortable with this idea, you can expand your conversations to include heart to heart woman talk, beyond the traditional mother/daughter roles.

@

Dad's been fondling himself lately. At home you gently guide him to his room while speaking to him in a calm and normal tone of voice:

"Dad, how about spending a little private time in your room?"

If it happens in public, take a deep breath before you quietly say to him,

"Dad, I think you should wait until we get home."

"What?"

"It's not really a good idea to touch yourself in public."

One day Dad reaches for you in an intimate way and calls you by your mother's name. You are horrified, but you pull yourself together and hold him at arm's length and say,

"Dad, I'd like to wait until after dinner for that hug. I appreciate it though."

He may be embarrassed if he realizes what he has done, but you can comfort him by taking his arm and saying,

"You must miss Mom very much. I know it's hard for you. I love you and I'm so glad you're here with me."

Ask him to take a break with you to enjoy some music and a chat about some of your favorite outings.

(Also: Dignity, Empathy, Privacy, Support Groups)

Personally I know nothing about sex because I've always been married.
-Zsa Zsa Gabor

SHARE CARE

Both you and Mom are going to need breaks from your daily routines as well as from each other. If you have family members living in the vicinity, ask for their assistance.

Review the sections in this book on respite care, senior centers, and day care. One other option you might consider is a novel concept we've chosen to call share care. It's a reasonable alternative to day care and senior centers and it doesn't have to cost you anything other than perhaps the cost of a movie or a meal.

Try connecting with other caregivers in your local Alzheimer's group or senior center. Periodically get together in small groups, two or three of you and your parents. Meet for a leisurely lunch at each other's homes, go to the movies together, or go out to dinner. It's a chance to develop social relationships for both you and your parent. But most importantly, it's also a great opportunity for you to generate a reliable network of caregivers who can cover for each other in emergency situations or if you need a break for an afternoon.

Please remember one ironclad rule: it's tempting to share your woes when you are out with this group of sympathetic people, but you all need to make an agreement ahead of time that any conversations about caregiving problems should be reserved for later telephone conversations away from your parents.

(Also: Comprehension, Day Care, Family, Respite, Support Groups)

Shared joy is a double joy; shared sorrow is half a sorrow.
- Swedish proverb

SIGNS

"CRASH!!!"

It's four o'clock in the morning. You're fast asleep when you're abruptly awakened by the sound of a crash coming from the living room. You fly out of bed in a panic, with visions of Dad lying on the floor with a broken leg. You run down the hallway toward the source of the noise, flipping on the overhead lights as you go. Dad's standing next to a shattered lamp, with a look of extreme urgency on his face. You guide him quickly into the bathroom, just in time.

The next day you go on a mission to make Dad's life (and yours) easier. Knowing that Dad still recognizes simple words, you put up a series of signs on the walls of your house. A "BATHROOM" sign, with an arrow pointing the way, is positioned in the hallway at eye level, another is placed just outside the kitchen, and finally a big one is posted on the door of the bathroom itself. Next, you put signs on Dad's room and the doors of other rooms, and you label such items as the laundry basket that Dad needs to identify. Don't panic: you don't have to do all of this in one day. You can make up, add, change, or replace signs as necessary.

The next step is to check the lighting in your house. Signs won't help if it's too dark for him to read them. You can introduce Dad to the signs you've made over the next few days by gently guiding him to each of them and reading them out loud. After several repetitions, it's likely he'll be able to follow them on his own.

Put a "STOP! DON'T GO OUT THIS DOOR!" on the inside of your exits and other doors that need to be secure.

Mom's vision isn't good so she often hangs a dress back in the closet, even if it's dirty. Doing the laundry was a major chore in Mom's youth and one did not wash a dress until it really needed it. You try to convince her that her dress should go in the wash, but she gets very upset.

"Mom, let's wash that dress."

"It's not dirty!"

"But Mom, you've worn it for the last three days in a row."

"Look at it: it's not dirty! There's no point in washing it; it's a waste of water."

"I have to wash all these other things in the hamper anyway, and there's enough space left over for your dress, so we're not using any extra water. Go ahead and put your dress in the hamper."

Mom peers down into the hamper at underwear and socks:

"I can't put my dress in there with those things!"

Before she gets upset again, you take the dress from her, careful to keep it separate from the other laundry as long as she's watching. Try putting a sign on the hamper: "ALL DIRTY CLOTHES GO HERE." If that doesn't work for Mom, buy a second plastic hamper for her dresses. Mark it: "DRESSES ONLY" and on the other: "OTHER DIRTY CLOTHES."

(Also: Home Safety, Obsessive Behavior, Wandering)

Things turn out best for people who make the best of the way things turn out.

                 -Anonymous

SINGING

Nobody in your family had much of an ear for music, so you're surprised when Mom starts to sing along with a radio station featuring oldies-but-goodies. To your amazement she recalls most of the lyrics and happily belts them out full blast and totally off key. You work up the nerve to hum along.

The car's a safe place for belting out old standards, on or off key. You may sound like a cat whose tail is slammed in a door, but who cares? You're having a good time and you're sharing some good laughs.

If Mom's mostly nonverbal, encouraging the grandchildren to sing along with her can create a special connection for them all. And besides, children can be generously forgiving of our imperfections and accept us just the way we are.

Your local library has music books galore and there are tapes and CDs on the market especially suitable for singalongs of oldies and goodies.

(Also: Children, Laughter, Music)

I think I should have no other mortal wants,
if I could always have plenty of music.
It seems to infuse strength into my limbs and
ideas into my brain. Life seems to go on with-
out effort, when I am filled with music.
- George Eliot

STRESS

You are, or you soon will be, an expert on stress! It's unavoidable to some degree, but there are things you can do to relieve and minimize the effects on you. Looking after Dad takes a lot of your energy, so you need to find ways to cope while keeping your own spirit up. Since he's so dependent on you, he will often reflect your moods and stress.

Try to maintain a balance between your own needs and his. Make time for a massage for yourself or an evening out with your friends. Continue to pursue your own interests and hobbies. When you plan activities to do with Dad, choose some that you'll enjoy as well. You can encourage Dad to help you make a wild sculpture or dig in the earth. Listening to soft music for relaxation or curling up with a good book can benefit both of you. If you have a dog or cat, you and Dad can spend time together, taking it for walks and grooming it. Cuddling a warm, fuzzy creature is tremendously calming.

Consider a yoga or stress management class for yourself. Don't forget the value of talking to others who are in the same situation. The importance of your Alzheimer's support group or a visit to a counselor or therapist could be invaluable in maintaining you sanity.

(Also: Counseling, Pets, Respite, Support Groups)

No pessimist ever discovered the secrets of the stars, or sailed to an uncharted land, or opened a new heaven to the human spirit.

-Helen Keller

SUNDOWNING

Mom tends to get restless at the same time every afternoon. She may be "sundowning." This term is used to describe agitation in some Alzheimer or dementia folks that occurs regularly in the late afternoon. It's believed to be a chemical reaction in the brain that's triggered by the waning light at the end of the day.

Her restlessness could be "sundowning" or simply a reaction to her old built-in body clock. A person who spends a lifetime doing a particular job with regular hours develops an internal clock that does not necessarily turn itself off at retirement. If Mom used to start dinner every day at 4 o'clock, it's natural for her to start getting anxious and fidgety at that time of day. Encourage her to help you with cooking or table-setting tasks.

@

You're told by the care facility Mom lives in that she is "sundowning." Before you take their word for it, find out if they have afternoon activities. Many residents are simply bored and frustrated from idleness that causes behavior similar to sundowning. Spend an afternoon at the home and if you suspect that her frustration is from boredom, talk to the management about establishing some afternoon activities.

You can also ask the staff to calm her down with a diversion. Give them some ideas. Suggest that they may tell her that she can relax because it's her day off and someone else is cooking dinner today. She may also calm down if they ask her to help set the tables or serve the water with dinner.

(Also: Diversions, Empathy, Kitchen, Music, Projects, Personal Space)

SUPPORT GROUPS

You might be doubting your caregiving skills as you face your daily challenges with Mom. We're recommending that you seek as much outside support as you can gather. First of all, ask your family to help you look after your mother. Caring for a person with Alzheimer's is an undertaking that needs to be shared by the whole family. Seek out one of the support groups sponsored by the Alzheimer's Association, and look into respite care, day care, and share care. Consider hiring a companion for Mom to take some of the load off your shoulders. You can also look into counseling for yourself so you'll have a safe outlet for expressing your feelings as well as a source for personal guidance.

◎

You have been regularly attending your local Alzheimer's Association support group meetings. There have been times when this group has been a real lifesaver for you. You've been able to share some of the uncomfortable feelings like guilt, resentment, and fear that you've found surfacing in you. It's reassuring to be able to share your anxieties and uncertainties with the other members. Lately, however, the meetings have turned into gripe sessions. You've come away with more negative feelings than positive ones.

A support group loses its effectiveness if it becomes a forum used solely to complain. How can you help the group make a turn-around?

Bring up the subject at the next meeting. It may be difficult, but it's likely that your feelings are shared by many of the others in the group. If they are receptive, explore together how the support group members can maintain a balance between expressing feelings and fears and helping each other find positive solutions to their particular challenges. It will help to share this book with everyone in the group.

If you find strong resistance to this discussion, it may not be the right group for you. You can seek out another Alzheimer's support group through the Alzheimer's Association. There are often several support groups in the same area, or you can start your own with folks you've met at the senior center.

(Also: Respite, Share Care)

The true test of character is not how much we know how to do, -
but how we behave when we don't know what to do.
-John Holt

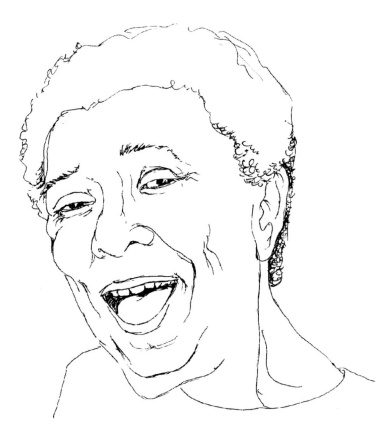

The ordinary tasks we practice every day at home are of more importance to the soul than their simplicity might suggest.

-Thomas Moore

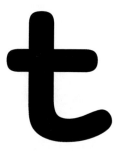

TELEPHONE

Since you moved away from home, you and your mother have stayed in touch with each other with frequent telephone calls. Lately you've had to do all the calling. When you reach Mom, she's profusely full of excuses that sound reasonable and sometimes she sounds surprised to hear your voice, although you've always talked to her before church on Sundays. Then one evening you return from work to find your telephone answering machine with seventeen messages on it; only two are not from Mom. You listen anxiously expecting a catastrophe, but she just sounds scared and confused about the answering machine itself, although she has used it confidently for years. On a couple of messages, she's crying. You immediately call her back, out of your mind with worry, and Mom is delighted to hear your voice. She's surprised and denies it when you mention the calls. She has no memory of calling you at all.

It has become apparent to you that Mom can no longer take care of herself, so you move her into your house without any hesitation. You and Mom have had such a close relationship all your adult life. It never crossed your mind to do anything different.

Your latest telephone bill shows a rather sizable charge for a couple dozen long distance calls to one number: your sister's answering machine. Your poor sister! And who knows, whom else Mom's been calling locally. She always loved to talk on the phone. Now that she's getting increasingly confused about it, she'll sometimes answer the phone politely and then immediately hang up on the caller. Lately she's become obsessive about talking to the same person she has just spoken to and calls her back as though for the first time.

The next time you see Mom reach for the phone again, you can gently intercept and cheerfully tell her about the wonderful conversation that she just had (even if it was in fact yesterday's conversation). Then you use one of your effective diversions:

"Mom, let's go in the kitchen and look at the catalog that arrived in the mail this morning. Maybe we can find a new pair of walking shoes for you."

When this no longer works, consider taking stronger measures, like keeping the phone out of sight inside a cabinet or drawer. If Mom discovers your ruse, you can unplug the phone until you're ready to use it and tell Mom that it's out of order. To be convincing, you may have to sound a little annoyed with the Phone Company.

"Things just aren't as reliable now as they were in the old days."

You can turn your answering machine's volume all the way down or get voice messaging service. Let family and friends know what the situation is, so they can call back if Mom hangs up on them or leave you messages on your voice-mail.

(Also: Diversions, Projects, Personal Space)

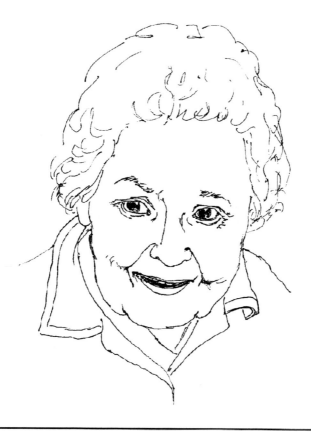

Well, if I called the wrong number,
why did you answer the 'phone?
-James Thurber

TELEVISION

Mom's been watching her soap opera faithfully for years, but one afternoon she becomes very agitated and is on the verge of tears. As far as you can tell, the story line is no different from the normal drama and tribulations of all the other episodes. You turn the sound down on the TV.

"Mom, what's happening? Why are you so upset?"

"She lost the baby, she lost the baby. Oh, it's terrible."

"Mom, she's an actress. She didn't really lose a baby. It's only make believe."

"But she just lost the baby."

There seems no way to soothe her right now. You fetch a tissue and wipe her tears.

"I'm really sorry about the baby. We can write her a card, okay? Would you like a glass of grape juice first?"

You realize that she may have trouble distinguishing between fact and fiction. From now on, you'll need to monitor her television viewing and watch any questionable material along with her. You may want to avoid watching the evening news, because of its graphic content. Looking at television through your mother's eyes, you'll find that much contemporary humor tends to be raunchy or mean-spirited and action programs may portray violence more graphically than she may be able to handle.

If Mom really enjoys the act of watching TV, you can invest in videos of special interest to her.

(Also: Comprehension, Movies, Reality, Videos)

TRANSITIONS

You've found a really good care facility for Mom, now that you've reached the stage in her dementia where it has become too difficult to care for her at home. Avoid discussing Mom's impending move too far in advance so that you don't cause her any unnecessary anxiety. You remember the trauma when she first came to live with you, so you're determined to do all you can to make her move into her new environment as easy and as stress-free as possible. You can make arrangements with the facility to take at least a couple of weeks to integrate Mom into her new home. Your goal is a gradual transition.

Make arrangements for you and Mom to eat at least a meal at the care facility two or three times a couple of weeks before her scheduled move. On you way there, talk with Mom as if it were just another outing:

"Mom, I thought we'd try a new place for lunch today. I hear it has good food and there are some really nice people there."

Then on the way home:

"I really enjoyed that lunch. The food was good, don't you think? And such nice people, especially that lady in the blue dress. She really liked you. You know, I'd like to go back again, wouldn't you?"

The second week, go to the facility every day, alternating between lunch and dinner. When you get home, continue to discuss your "new favorite place."

During the last two weeks before her move, join Mom in participating in some of the facility's activity programs. In addition, encourage her to spend more time visiting with her future roommates. At this point you can introduce the idea that it would be a good place to live:

"Mom, we have to get going now, but it sure would be so nice to spend more time here, don't you think?"

Consider all the variations of this approach and then increasingly build on the idea of living there:

"I'm sorry we had to leave so soon. I know you'd like to spend more time with your friends, wouldn't you? You know, they really like you and they seem sad every time you have to leave. I wonder if they might have a room there for you. Wouldn't that be great? Then you'd be close to your friends all the time. We can ask, right? Cross your fingers."

And then finally, the day before her move, be really excited:

"Oh Mom, I have the best news for you! I just got a phone call and they saved one of their best rooms for you. Isn't that exciting? I told them that you'd be very happy to hear that. We'd better jump on it before they give it to someone else. Come on, let's celebrate!"

On moving day, take her to the facility in the morning and let her mingle with her friends while you discreetly move her belongings into her room. Be sure her pictures and possessions are in place before you bring her to it. Walk her in as if it were a the executive suite at a four star hotel:

"Welcome to your room, Mom. Boy, aren't we lucky that this was available? Isn't it nice? Look at this great view (if it has one) and see how lovely your pictures look in here."

Sit down with her in her new place and have a normal and casual conversation. She will see how comfortable you feel being there and that will help her get over any possible anxiety. Stay with her until her bedtime and try to have breakfast with her the following morning.

During the next few weeks, join her for as many meals and activities as you can. You can gradually taper off to a reasonable number of visits. It's very important to let her know that you want to spend time with her there and that you'll continue to do so.

It sounds like a lot of work, and it is, but taking the time now will save you the stress you'd no doubt go through if Mom was moved in without any preparation at all.

(Also: Care Facilities, Empathy, Environment, Guilt)

Maybe one of these days I'll be able to give myself a gold star for being ordinary,

and maybe one of these days I'll give myself a star for being extraordinary – for persisting.

And maybe one day I won't need a star at all.

-Sue Bender

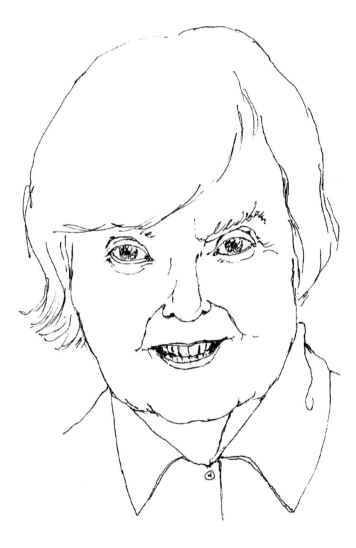

Difficult times have helped me to understand better than before how infinitely rich and beautiful life is in every way and that so many things that one goes worrying about are of no importance whatsoever.

-Isak Dinesen

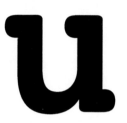

UNDRESSING

Dad walks into the dining room without a stitch of clothing on. You gasp in shock, trying not to react in disapproval. This is unthinkable! You were raised to be modest. Dad's nudity is so shocking that you have no idea how to handle it.

Take a very deep breath and say as casually as you can:

"Hi, Dad. Looks as if you couldn't decide what to wear. Come on, let's go to your room and we'll find you a really nifty outfit for today."

Or:

"It's a little cold tonight. I think we should find you some clothes to put on. What would you like to wear today, your dark blue sweats? Or your beige slacks and the brown shirt we bought last week?"

Chances are that he will cooperate with you and let you help him. There's likely a good reason for his nudity. He could simply have forgotten how to get dressed or how to get to his clothes in his closet. He may be too hot. If it's not a hot summer's day, he may be running a temperature and this may be the only way for him to tell you that something is wrong.

If he seems well and simply does not want to get dressed, what's the harm of nudity at home?

If you have a persistent problem with Dad's undressing, especially in public, think about buying him specialty clothing that is difficult for him to remove without your help. You can buy him jumpsuits with closures in the back so he can't get out of them by himself, but remember that you'll have to help him whenever he needs to use the toilet. If you have a sewing machine, you can alter some of the garments he already wears by stitching closed the front plackets of a shirt and sewing a long zipper into the back. If you want to get elaborate, sew top and bottom together and install a very long zipper in the back. Sweats lend themselves well to this alteration.

(Also: Coaching, Dignity, Reactions)

Love is a little blind; when we love someone dearly we unconsciously overlook many faults.
-Beatrice Saunders

V

VIDEOS

Sundays at your parents' house typically would be Mom and the women in the kitchen or garden; Dad and the men in the den glued to the television set. He still enjoys watching football games, but increasingly he gets so involved in the conflict that he carries his anger into the rest of the day. As far as you can tell his dementia is causing a distortion of his perceptions of what he sees; he has a hard time following the game, separating the outbursts and even getting commercials confused with the game.

For a while you've been watching the games with Dad to have the opportunity to talk him through some of the rough spots. You've never been a football fan and he gets upset at your ignorance.

You're looking for a way to keep both of you content. One suggestion: videos.

You can acquire videos of NFL highlights and NFL bloopers, maybe a Super Bowl or two. Dad can watch these videos repeatedly and, because they're familiar, chances are that he will not become agitated.

It's not just football that causes Dad stress. You've noticed that he has difficulty distinguishing fiction from reality in a lot of his favorite television dramas. You are taking the precaution of viewing these shows with him, so you reiterate to him that his watching make-believe.

Videos are a good alternative since you can't always be with him. Almost any topic is available on video: architecture to zebras, Humphrey Bogart to Sid Caesar. Check with your local library and video stores. You might also consider taping Dad's favorite television shows to play back at times better suited to his schedule. If Dad was a movie fan in his youth, you might consider owning a collection of classics for him. Look on the Internet for web sites that specialize in classic movies. It may be a major investment for you, but worth it if Dad is happy spending hours looking at his old favorites. He may not be able to follow the story line too well, especially on the small screen, but chances are that he knows it by heart anyway. Besides, just watching his favorite actors is probably pleasure enough for him. Many of the larger video rental stores have a sizable collection of the classics or are willing to order them for you.

(Also: Movies, Television)

If people did not sometimes do silly things, nothing intelligent would ever get done.
-Wittgenstein

VISITORS

Your brother's coming to visit from out of state for the first time in a few years. Mom has been quite confused lately and chances are that she won't recognize him. You want to initiate their reunion with care, especially for your brother's sake. He has come a long way with high expectations and will likely be hurt if the visit does not well.

Before you take your brother in to see Mom, meet with him to help him make this a successful encounter. You explain to him about communicating with Mom. Have him read the section on "Memories" in this book and reiterate with him the pitfalls of "Do you remember . . .?" questions.

Tell him that Mom has a strong adverse reaction to patronizing baby talk and remind him to keep his tone moderate, but adult. Make it clear to him that Mom understands a lot more than her appearance would suggest.

You told Mom last night and again this morning that her son's coming.

"I have a surprise for you, Mom. Your son, John, is coming for a visit. I'm really looking forward to seeing my brother, and because it's been such a long time since he was last here, I wonder if we'll recognize him. He may look very different now."

Mom doesn't handle surprise very well, so you'll have to ease your brother back into her awareness. You've let him know ahead of time how you intend to introduce him and ask him to wait for your cue before he talks to Mom. As you walk him up to meet her, you say in a calm and cheerful voice:

"Mom, I want you to meet this handsome young man. Believe it or not, this is your son, John. John, this is your beautiful mother. I'm so lucky that she's living here with me. We have such a good time together."

If she does not react, keep talking to her in an adult tone of voice and gesture to John to do the same.

"Well, John, I bet Mom would like to hear how you're doing these days. Wouldn't you, Mom? Do you still have that interesting job?"

And later:
"We have some good news for you, John. Mom and I have found a new hairdresser. That may not mean a whole lot to you with your short hair, but we really like to go see her. She's a nice person and she's good."

Mom doesn't have to say a word to feel part of the conversation. You assume that Mom comprehends every word. If your brother forgets and starts talking about her as though she can't hear, you can bail him out by redirecting his question to Mom:

"Mom, John's asking you if your back's still bothering you. What do you say? To me, it seems to have improved so much that you've forgotten all about it."

With your help, your brother's visit can be fulfilling and fun for all of you. Mom may forget the event almost immediately, but chances are the good feelings will stay with her.

(Also: Communication, Conversations, Memories)

VITAMINS

Many elderly folks just don't eat enough and may be suffering from vitamin deficiencies. Malnutrition, dehydration, and vitamin deficiencies are often found in those suffering from cognitive disorders, such as Alzheimer's disease and dementia. Some of these causes are reversible, but even if the damage has already been done, it doesn't hurt to do everything in your power to slow down further deterioration.

As we age, our bodies' ability to absorb vitamins decreases. Even if you eat a healthy diet, you can still be lacking certain crucial nutrients.

Folate (folic acid) appears to be the one B vitamin that's most crucial to brain health. Studies are suggesting that folate deficiencies aggravate brain lesions in Alzheimer's. Government research estimates that 80% of Americans fall short of the recommended daily minimum of 400 micrograms. The best natural sources of folic acid are legumes, green leafy vegetables (especially spinach,) citrus fruit, and whole grain products.

Antioxidants help combat free radicals. Antioxidants are found naturally in fresh fruit and vegetables, as well as green and black teas. Antioxidants are vitamins C, E, and B.

Free radicals are unstable oxygen molecules, which can damage healthy cell membranes and tissue. Free radicals have been implicated in cancer, heart disease, Alzheimer's, and many other physical conditions.

Vitamin Supplements

It is very hard to obtain enough of these critical vitamins through diet alone, especially for the elderly. You will want to supplement Dad's diet. Look for a reliable brand of commercial multivitamins especially formulated for the elderly and talk to his doctor about adding extra beta-carotene, calcium, vitamins A, C, D3, and vitamin E (recognized as an especially important component in combating Alzheimer's progression.)

Many vitamin tablets are so large that they may be hard for Dad to swallow, in which case you can purchase a liquid vitamin or you can crush them and mix them with a little jelly.

(Also: Alternative Remedies, Alzheimer's Disease, Dementia, Diet, Medication, Pills)

Good instincts usually tell you what to do before your head has figured it out.
            -Michael Burke

W

WALKING

Mom walks very cautiously these days. She slows down and seems to "feel" her way with the toe of her shoe. You recently had her vision tested and it seems reasonably normal, so her confusion must be caused by her dementia. Because of her problems you've been paying particular attention to how you yourself move about. You've noticed that you routinely survey and register what's ahead of you as you walk. You unconsciously "memorize" the path ahead. With that idea in mind, Mom's behavior makes perfect sense. She has trouble with abstract concepts and remembering in general, so it's no wonder she has difficulty with walking. She can't memorize the terrain.

Get into the habit of acting as Mom's eyes and memory by engaging in a descriptive commentary of walking as you hold her by the arm:

"A curb coming up, Mom. Then it's smooth for a while."

As you tap your toe at the edge of the first step, you say,

"We're going down three steps now. Here's the first one."

"We'll go around the corner up ahead. It's a little uneven, but there are no steps."

You're thinking out loud for both of you with your descriptive commentary. Before long this behavior will be so ingrained in you that you may find yourself doing it with your friends.

This is the best and safest way to hold Mom's arm while you walk with her:

Bend the elbow of your arm and hold Mom's arm, also bent at the elbow close to your side. Clasp her hand lightly and hold her so her elbow is resting against your waist. Should she stumble, you have a firm and safe hold on her through the entire length of her arm, which will keep her upright without much of a ripple and with risk of injury at a minimum.

It's important that you not lace your fingers with Mom's. Should you need to move quickly to grab her, you'd be slowed down by having to unlace them.

This "hold" not only keeps Mom stable on her feet, it also keeps the two of you side by side, making your conversations more connected and intimate. It helps Mom feel equal to you. Avoid dragging or leading her behind you because you won't be able to see how she's moving along. It's also an impatient maneuver, similar to the way many of us used to drag our kids around when they were walking too slowly. It's inconsiderate to treat our children or Mom in this manner.

(Also: Body Language, Coaching)

WANDERING

One morning while still dressed in her pajamas, Mom decides to take a walk by herself. You had gone to the bathroom for just a moment, yet when you return to the living room, the front door is wide open and Mom's nowhere to be seen. A quick glance up and down the street reveals nothing. You jump in the car and drive around the block, imagining the worst, of course — and then there she is, petting a miniature poodle, looking as happy as a clam. You are so relieved and at the same time you want to scream at her for putting you through this trauma. Many of us have yelled in fear at our young children for running into the street after a ball. Anger is a natural reaction to fear.

As you climb out of the car, you take a deep breath and join her as she continues to visit with the dog. Take your time until you're calm again, then gently guide her back to the car, nodding a smile to any curious neighbors looking on. Once you've her into the car, you can try to talk to her about what happened. She may be able to understand, but on the other hand, if she doesn't hear you, try a different approach:

"It sure is a beautiful day today, a great day to be outside. I can understand why you wanted to go for a walk. I'd love to come with you next time. How about this? First we'll go home and finish our breakfast and then we can plan the rest of the day. We can go out for a walk together later today if you like. Okay?"

You have some decisions and preparations to make now, because you know this will happen again. Is there a way to secure your home exits without feeling like a prisoner yourself?

In the city, you can enlist the help of your neighbors and alert them to the possibility of Mom's wandering. You can distribute a flyer (see Neighborhood Flyer) with Mom's picture and description around your neighborhood so that people will be informed of Mom's condition.

౨౦

You may face different problems if you live in a rural area. You may have to enclose your surrounding yard or garden with a secure fence. Should Mom manage to wander off in spite of all your precautions, alert your local search and rescue team right away. Mom could easily get lost in the desert or woods and suffer from exposure or hypothermia.

The search for Mom may be challenging. Because of her confusion, she can become very creative in her exploring, so her wandering might not necessarily be logical. She may have decided to go "home," meaning back to her childhood when things were simple and safe. If she has that idea in mind, it's natural for her to play "hide and seek," "cops and robbers," or "treasure hunt." She's probably not even aware that she's "lost." As far as she's concerned, she has a definite purpose and destination.

Get Mom a Medical Alert bracelet. We recommend that you have it inscribed with "Alzheimer's." Mom may not have Alzheimer's disease, but it's the most recognized term for dementia-related conditions.

Visit your local police department and hospital emergency rooms. Give them a packet of information that includes a current picture of Mom and relevant information about her.

(Also: Identification, Conversations, Neighborhood Flyer, Safe Return)

WORD GAMES

Even if Mom's verbal skills are not too adept any more, there are certain things she can still recall, with a little prodding from you. Proverbs, platitudes, and old sayings often stay in our memories longer than personal experiences. Games provide good stimulation when they are approached as a shared and playful experience. Avoid competitiveness or putting anyone on the spot. Play only as long as it's fun for both of you and remember the most important factor is the socialization that happens. Many of these games work especially well in a group, so introduce them to your share care group or try them at a family gathering.

Name Game

Select a four or five-letter word or name.

Take the name RITA as an example. Think of three girl's names and three boy's names starting with the letter "R," the letter "I," then "T," and finally "A."

"Rose, Ruth, and Renee;" "Isabel, Iris, and Irene;" "Tommy, Ted, and Tim," or "Adam, Amos, and Alan," for example.

Keep the pace brisk and go on to the next letter if there's a lull. This is a great game as long as it's treated as fun and not a chore or competition.

If a certain name brings up memories for Mom, go with her flow and encourage her to reminisce as much as she likes. Keep your journal or tape recorder handy in case Mom shares some new gems from her memory bank.

Naming Things

Car brands, states of the union, presidents, TV shows, writers, animals, countries, occupations, holidays, etc.

Vegetables, fruits, ice creams, desserts, sandwiches, drinks.

Make up a menu for a picnic, a party, or a flight to the moon. Make up weird combinations: strawberry pizza, hamburger pudding, asparagus with chocolate syrup, etc.

Platitudes

This is a fun game for just the two of you. See how long you can keep it going. You take turns coming up with a platitude or cliche:

"How are you doin'?"

"As well as can be, how's about you?"

"Hanging in there!"

"You sound peachy."

"Oh, it's hunky dory."

"So you're in the pink?"

"Could be worse."

"Well, tomorrow is another day."

"One day is like another.

"Easy come, easy go."

Etc.

Proverbs and Sayings
You'll probably be amazed how much Mom remembers. We give you a few samples and suggest that you start a collection of your own.

Start the proverb and let Mom or the group finish it.

Home, sweet (home)

By hook or (by crook)

A penny saved is a (penny earned)

A bird in the hand is worth (two in the bush)

There's no place like (home)

An apple a day keeps (the doctor away)

An onion a day keeps (everybody away)

In one ear (out the other)

It's better to be safe than (sorry)

If the shoe fits (wear it)

Don't cry over (spilt milk)

Where there's smoke there's (fire)

When the cat's away (the mice will play)

Necessity is the mother of (invention)

It's as plain as the nose on (your face)

For crying out (loud)

Action speaks louder than (words)

Don't put all your eggs in (one basket)

Strike while the iron is (hot)

He's a fish out of (water)

He's got a skeleton in the (closet)

Beggars can't be (choosers)

Practice makes (perfect)

Between the devil and the (deep blue sea)

It's like taking candy from (a baby)

You can't teach an old dog (new tricks)

A rolling stone gathers (no moss)

Better late than (never)

It takes two to (tango)

Easy come, easy (go)

Heavens to (Betsy)

You can lead a horse to water, (but you can't make him drink)

Story Making

This game can be played with a group of people or just the two of you. Go as fast you can, giving your first reactions. You'll end up with a nonsensical story, which makes this game so much fun. Write it down, so you can share it when you've finished.

For example:

"Once upon a time there was a . . .?"

"crocodile."

"He lived in a . . .?"

"Brooklyn Bridge."

"His favorite pastime was to . . .?"

"read". . .

And so on . . .

Word Twister

Try this game in a group and let it flow naturally. Food is an easy topic, because everyone can relate to it. It might go like this:

"What's your favorite pie?"

"Apple!"

"What else do we make with apple?"

"Jelly!"

"What other kind of jelly do we eat?"

"Strawberry!"

"What else do we make with strawberry?"

"Ice cream!"

"Hey, how about a strawberry ice cream break right now?"

(Also: Games, Humor, Laughter, Projects, Personal Space)

Could we change our attitude, we should not only see life differently, but life itself would come to be different. Life would undergo a change of appearance because we ourselves had undergone a change of attitude.
-Katherine Mansfield

WORD SUBSTITUTIONS

"I want more grun on my cereal"

Dad's losing his grasp of language and has started substituting words for those he's forgotten. Most of the time it's easy to interpret what he means.

"Would you like more milk on your cereal, Dad?"

"That's what I said!"

If you suspect you know what Dad means by his substitution, use the accurate word in your response, but avoid making it sound like a correction. If you have no idea what on earth he's talking about, let your response be vague and interested enough to solicit a second remark from him. Bit by bit you'll piece it together. He says,

"Where's the green?"

Does he mean green shirt? Or does "green" mean something else entirely, like "dog," "toothbrush," or the Mozart CD? You need more to go on.

"I don't recall seeing it lately, I wonder if it could be outside."

"Of course not, Stupid! I just mooed it."

"I'll help you look, Dad. Was it the big one or the little one?"

"My green!" as he picks up a half-eaten sandwich.

He may use substitutions randomly or he may have one favorite word that he uses for anything of importance. It can be tempting to use these substitutions yourself, but try to resist. Remember that he's probably trying to find the correct word in his head, so using his substitute word may confuse or insult him.

"I want to wear the blue loyal today." (= shirt)

"You look so good in the blue shirt, Dad."

"I'm going to read my loyal now." (=book)

"I have heard it's a very good book. How do you like it?"

"I am so loyal now." (=tired or hungry?)

"I am hungry and tired, too. I'll fix us some lunch now, and then we can take a nap afterwards. Sound good to you?"

You knew he meant either hungry or tired, so with this response you have given him both.

(Also: Communications, Conversations, Discussions, No!, Questions)

If you are patient in one moment, you will escape a hundred days of sorrow.

-Chinese proverb

Love cures people – both the ones who give it and the ones who receive it.

-Karl Menninger

APPENDIX

Books

36 Hour Day
A Family Guide to Caring for Persons with Alzheimer's Disease, Related Demeaning Illnesses, and Memory Loss in Later Life
by Nancy L. Mace, M.A. and Peter V. Rabins, M.D., M.P.H.
Publisher: Warner Books

The Complete Guide to Alzheimer's Proofing Your Home
by Mark Warner, A.I.A.
Publisher: Ageless Design

How I Find Her
by Genie Zeiger
Publisher: Sherman Asher

Caregiving: The Spiritual Journey of Love, Loss, and Renewal
by Beth Witrogen McLeod
Publisher: John Wiley & Sons

Decoding Darkness
The Search for the Genetic Causes of Alzheimer's Disease
by Rudolph E. Tanzi and Ann B. Parson
Publisher: Perseus Publishing

Prescription for Nutritional Healing
A Practical A-Z Reference to Drug-Free Remedies Using Vitamins, Minerals, Herbs & Food Supplements
By James F. Balch, M.D., Phyllis A. Balch, C.N.C.
Publisher: Avery Publishing Group

Worst Pills, Best Pills
A Consumer's Guide to Avoiding Drug-induced Death or Illness
by Sidney M. Wolfe, Editor, Larry D. Sasich, Rose-Ellen Hope
Publisher: Public Citizen

Support Groups

The Alzheimer's Association National Office
919 North Michigan Avenue, Suite 1000
Chicago, IL 60611-1676
(800) 272-3900
(312) 335-8700
Fax: (312) 335-1110

The Alzheimer's Association is a national group with numerous local chapters. Call the toll free number listed to contact your local affiliation. Most chapters offer support groups that can be a good place to connect to people with whom you establish a share-care group. If there isn't a chapter close to you, ask the Association for assistance in establishing one in your area.

National Institute on Aging, National Institutes of Health
7550 Wisconsin Ave., Rm 618
Bethesda, MD 20892
(301) 496-5345
Brochures on Alzheimer's and dementia and information on programs for the elderly.

National Hospice Organization
1901 N. Moore St., Suite 901
Arlington, VA 22209
(703) 243-5900

Ombudsman's Program
Administration on Aging
330 Independence Ave. SW
Washington, DC 20201

The Ombudsman's program has a federal mandate to act as advocates for residents of nursing homes and care facilities. This office is a good resource for local programs and facilities. Contact the Administration on Aging at the above address or look in your yellow pages under United States government, Agency on Aging.

Senior Centers

Most towns have at least one senior center. Look for stimulating programs such as dancing, arts and crafts and special movies. This is another good source for participants in a share-care group.

Local Hospitals

Many hospitals now have special group sessions for people with Alzheimer's and dementia. If Dad's able, encourage him to participate. Usually run by a social worker or therapist, this group can give him emotional support. This is especially helpful if he's in the early stages of Alzheimer's and needs answers to his many questions about his condition or if he suffers from anxieties.

Information

Alzheimer's web pages:
www.agelessdesign.com
www.Susan@alzwell.com
www.elderweb.com

Care Facility Information
www.consumerreports.org
(Shopping for a Nursing Home)

ADEAR
Alzheimer's Disease Education and Referral Center
P.O. Box 8250
Silver Spring, MD 20907-8250
(800) 438-4380
www.adear@alzheimers.org

National Institute on Aging
Public Information Office
Building 31, Room 5C27
31 Center Drive, MSC 2292
Bethesda, MD 20892
(301) 496-1752

National Council on Aging
409 Third St. SW
Washington, DC 20024
(202) 479-1200

Legal information:
www.nolo.com

Products

AARP
(Request their home care catalog)
3557 Lafayette Rd.
Indianapolis, IN 46272
email:member@aarp.org

Buck & Buck Designs
Specialty clothing
3111 27th Avenue South
Seattle, WA 98144-6502
(800) 458-0600

J. C. PENNEY
Catalog: Special Needs
Home health care products
(800) 222-6161

S&S Healthcare
(800) 243-9232
Great resource for all kinds of crafts kits, games, and hobby supplies.

SEARS, Shop at Home
Home Health Care
(800) 733-7249

Wardrobe Wagon Specialty clothing
Call for free catalog (800) 992-2737
info@wardrobewagon.com

Identification
Ask your local pharmacist or contact:

American Medical Identifications
P.O. Box 925512
Houston, TX 77292
(800) 363-5985

medical-id.com (gold and silver)
P.O. Box 50
Verbank, NY 12585
(800) 830-0546

Medic Alert
2323 Colorado
Turlock, CA 95381-9009
(800) 825-3785

Safe Return
(Alzheimer's Association program)
(888) 572-8566 or (800) 272-3900

Movies, Videos, Music
www.amazon.com
www.bestvideo.com
www.blockbuster.com
or 1(800)441-4736
www.nationalgeographic.com
www.pbs.org
www.reel.com

And for you:
Complaints of a Dutiful Daughter
A film by Deborah Hoffman
Distributed by "Women Make Movies"

ABOUT YOUR AUTHOR

Jytte Lokvig

Jytte Lokvig, BA, MA, combines her lifelong passions as an artist and educator. She was a member of the original staff of a pilot program that has since become the model for the current magnet schools in Los Angeles, California.

For nearly a decade Jytte has turned her energies to working with the elderly, especially those with Alzheimer's disease and related dementia. Her personal experiences and clinical research have shown that active involvement in the world is crucially important to emotional life and health, particularly for those with these debilitating disorders.

Jytte designs and implements activities that combine her expertise in arts, theater, and music with her background in educational psychology, resulting in an environment filled with joyful exploration. Her focus is on enhancing the quality of life for those individuals who cannot speak and do for themselves. She says, "The approach I'm using now with the elderly is quite similar to what I used as a teacher of young people. I encourage those experiences I consider essential to the survival of the human spirit. These activities promote self-respect, exploration, and creative expression."

This book is a drawn from Jytte's years of experience as well as her work in counseling families.

Let Us Hear From You

This book was written for you, the caregiver, to help you with your daily experiences. We've tried to discuss most of the kinds of situations that you may encounter, but we're aware that it is impossible to cover everything for everybody. Therefore we invite you to contact us with your questions, concerns, anecdotes, or comments.

Overall Rating

Hated it   OK   Loved it
  1 _____ 2 _____ 3 _____ 4 _____ 5

What I liked best about this book:

This is the section or idea that helped me the most:

Here are my suggestions for improvements:

This is what I think you should add to the next edition:

Other comments:

I have been a caregiver since:

My favorite moment as caregiver:

My biggest frustration:

My most effective diversion:

My most effective approach at bath time:

I could use some ideas with this situation:

Optional:

Name_____

Phone number _____

e-mail address (for our use only) _____

Mail this to:
Alzheimer's A to Z
228 Ojo de la Vaca
Santa Fe, NM 87508

Or e-mail us:
AlzheimersAtoZ@cs.com

ORDER FORM

Alzheimer's A to Z
228 Ojo de la Vaca
Santa Fe, NM 87508

Phone orders: (505)466-8195 or (575)466-8195
e-mail: AlzheimersAtoZ@cs.com

___Soft Cover @ $19.95   _____
Shipping and handling:
$4.50 first item, $2.00 each additional item _____
                                      $_____

Name _____

Address _____

City _____ State ____ Zip _____

Telephone number   (   ) _____

e-mail _____

Payment: ☐ Check   ☐ Moneyorder

☐ Master Card   ☐ Visa   ☐ Discover   ☐ AMEX

Card number _____

Name on card _____ Exp. date _____

ORDER FORM
Alzheimer's A to Z
228 Ojo de la Vaca
Santa Fe, NM 87508

Phone orders: (505)466-8195 or (575)466-8195
e-mail: AlzheimersAtoZ@cs.com

___Soft Cover @ $19.95   _____
Shipping and handling:
$4.50 first item, $2.00 each additional item _____
                                                    $_____

Name _____

Address _____

City _____ State ____ Zip _____

Telephone number   (   ) _____

e-mail _____

Payment: ☐ Check   ☐ Moneyorder

☐ Master Card   ☐ Visa   ☐ Discover   ☐ AMEX

Card number _____

Name on card _____ Exp. date _____